A Short Good Life

A Short Good Life

*Her Father Tells Liza's Story
of Facing Death*

PHILIP LISTER

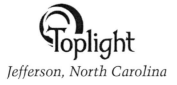

Toplight

Jefferson, North Carolina

Author's note: Several names have been changed for privacy.

ISBN (print) 978-1-4766-8557-1
ISBN (ebook) 978-1-4766-4344-1

LIBRARY OF CONGRESS AND BRITISH LIBRARY
CATALOGUING DATA ARE AVAILABLE

Library of Congress Control Number 2021037332

Front cover: Photograph of Liza in the summer of 1994 (Philip Lister)

Printed in the United States of America

Toplight is an imprint of McFarland & Company, Inc., Publishers

Box 611, Jefferson, North Carolina 28640
www.toplightbooks.com

TABLE OF CONTENTS

But we need books that affect us like a disaster, that grieve us deeply, like the death of someone we loved more than ourselves.... A book must be the axe for the frozen sea within us.

~ Franz Kafka

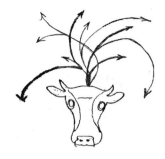

Introduction:
The Wonderful World
of Color
2019

Liza first cherished red and blue as her favorite colors when she was one year old. Molly, three years older, showed her how to make purple for the first time. When she saw that red and blue combined to make purple, purple displaced red and became Liza's favorite, along with blue.

We have a video of our family in our living room during a visit from my mother when Liza was two. Molly asked with a chuckle, "Lizie, what is your favorite color?"

Liza replied, as Molly knew she would, hamming to the camera, "Berry, berry, berry, berry, berry, berry, berry dark blue!"

Liza hadn't yet gotten the *v* sound in "very." But I had to write this as "berry" rather than "bery" because of something that happened in the Berkshires.

We were vacationing there, and we stopped in the woods to go blueberry picking. My wife, Elena, and I both carried bowls, and the girls toted plastic buckets. Liza couldn't seem to get the hang of putting a berry into the bucket. They all went into her mouth instead. Within twenty-four hours, with no distress, her diaper was berry, berry, berry dark blue indeed.

1

We vacationed in the Berkshires several summers in a row. Elena and I, both psychiatrists, took vacations in August, like many of our colleagues. The last summer, we stayed in a house with a heated pool. In her pink and purple one-piece, intrepid Molly raced me or Elena the length of the pool, scrambled out and onto the diving board, and then jumped back in what seemed like hundreds of times. Liza wore a royal-blue suit with a ring of Styrofoam blocks in slots all the way around her midsection, which kept her afloat. Entranced by her sister, Liza paddled around quickly, coming to trust the buoyancy of the foam, unconcerned with her feet touching bottom. After watching a bunch of Molly's jumps, Liza hopped in from the side of the pool. A little braver each time, she started jumping from the diving board just like her big sister. Eventually, Elena would go inside to start dinner, and when she gave the shout that it was ready, we bundled ourselves in towels and headed to a collective shower to warm up.

With Elena navigating, I drove our rental car through the countryside, and we would all sing along to CDs of Raffi or Laurie Berkner. Sometimes the girls would start giggling on their own, or I would get them giggling by making faces into the rearview mirror. Then Elena or I would declare, with mock sternness, "No laughing in this car! Stop that giggling right now!"

Over the summer days, that injunction evolved so that the girls would dish it back to us. "Mommy and Daddy, stop that chuckling! Don't you know there is no chuckling in this car?" Then we would feign crying, in protest to the unfair treatment they were imposing.

Soon these became short directives from the backseat: "Laugh, Mommy and Daddy!" and then "Now cry, Daddy! Cry, Mommy!" They delighted at our lurching emotional repertoire, all at their command.

Liza, quietly, would catch my eye in the mirror. She'd scrunch up her face as if nearly blinded by the sun. It always made me laugh, and so she realized she held this power over me. Sometimes when we were walking down the street, she would pull back. When I'd turn around to see what held her up, she'd give me the scrunched-up face that always cracked me up.

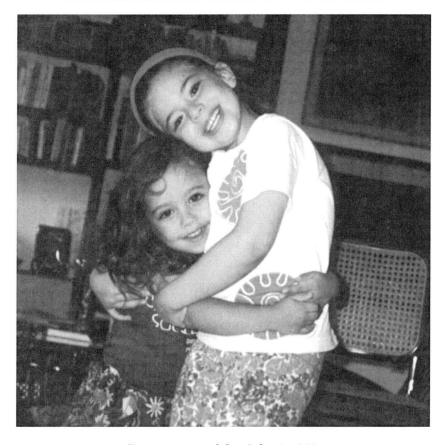

Sisters on a good day, July 31, 1993.

Other times she could be impossibly stubborn. Once when she was two, I asked her to get dressed. She complied but had trouble getting her shoes on. She was trying to put the right shoe on the left foot.

"It goes on the other foot, Lizie," I explained.

"No, it doesn't," she said. "I just can't get it on."

"We need to get out of here, Liza. Let me help you."

"No, Daddy, I can do it." After another minute, she was tripping with the shoes partway on the wrong feet.

The next thing I remember is that I had her pinned to the ground, jamming the shoes onto the correct feet. She screamed the whole time.

When it came to toilet training, she was equally hardheaded, showing no willingness to part from her beloved diapers. Force was useless, of course. But there was a shop near our home, and we noticed that Liza was entranced by the big red dinosaur in its window.

After a little scheming, Elena and I walked slowly by the shop with Liza one afternoon and paused. As Liza ogled the stuffed brontosaurus bigger than she was, I turned to her. "Lizie, would you like to earn the dinosaur?"

Her eyes widened. "Really? Yes!"

"Well, if you're ready to give up your diapers, we'll get it for you."

"I want to!"

"Let's see if you can go ten days with no diapers, and when you can, we'll come back and get the red dinosaur for you."

And that's what happened.

I think I loved that dinosaur as much as she did.

PART I

All the Way to the Deep End

October 1994–September 1995

When you are sorrowful look again in your heart, and you shall see that in truth you are weeping for that which has been your delight.

~ Kahlil Gibran

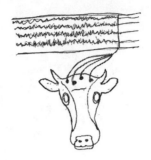

1—Bone Marrow Biopsy

October 1994

It's autumn in New York City, and Liza is four years old. For three weeks, she has felt under the weather. She has had low-grade fevers and aches and pains that have wandered from hip to shoulder to sinuses. After the second complaint, she received some antibiotics. After the third, she had a blood test. One result was extremely abnormal, and more tests were required at the emergency department. When none of them were conclusive, the doctors scheduled a bone marrow biopsy.

On Monday morning, October 31, after the weekend at home, we go to Mount Sinai Hospital's pediatric clinic. Through a maze of corridors, we find our way to a dark waiting room. A nurse walking by, her face painted with a doggy nose and whiskers, assures us this is the right place and turns on the lights.

My mother, Charlotte, has rushed up from Baltimore, my hometown, over the weekend, and she has come with us to the hospital. She is a stylish, short, spry woman who turned seventy last summer. Though the soberness of the occasion shows on her face, she is wearing whimsical, multicolored earrings that dangle like miniature Calders. They complement her cocked, wide-brimmed gold hat. She has spent more time with us since my father died five years ago. With Charlotte here, Elena and I can be alone with the doctors when that's necessary, while Nanny (as our kids call her) keeps Liza company. Her older sister, seven-year-old Molly, is at school today in first grade.

Dr. Arthur Stevens comes to us, greets Liza, meets my mom, and then escorts Elena and me to one of the small examining rooms. Here he takes shape: a balding, slim man with wire-rimmed glasses, small blue eyes, a short brown beard. I am struck by his kind voice and face, as I had been when first meeting him. Dr. Lisa Mueller joins us. Dr. Stevens discusses the plan to do the bone marrow biopsy now, allowing for a definitive diagnosis.

"How long will it take to get the results?" I ask.

"It will take some hours to evaluate the biopsy material."

"Can we leave and have the day at home?" Elena wants to know. "Even keep our evening plans for trick-or-treating?"

As soon as results are ready, the doctors assure us, they'll beep me on my pager. If the suspected diagnosis is confirmed, we will return tomorrow morning for Liza to be admitted to the hospital for treatment.

"Which of you wants to be with Liza for the procedure?" Dr. Stevens asks.

"I do," Elena and I both answer without hesitation. He pauses for a moment, and I sense what he's considering. Should he agree to let us both be there or refuse and force us to choose?

After a moment, he says, "Okay. As physicians, you know what procedures of this kind are like. But if either of you gets upset, nurses will be there to hold her, and you should feel no shame if you need to leave the room." Tacitly, he acknowledges that as long as we remain calm, Liza will be more comfortable with us beside her.

I ask, "Who will do the procedure?" wondering if it will be Dr. Stevens, the attending, or Dr. Mueller, the fellow.

Dr. Stevens answers, "Dr. Mueller will do it." In a manner Elena and I remember all too well from our own medical training, he adds, "She has done many more of these procedures recently than I have." The line of reasoning is all too familiar as well—logical, but totally unsettling. Just because she has done more procedures recently, does she really do them better than, or even as well as, the more experienced attending? Dr. Mueller seems so young, so green, while Dr. Stevens seems so capable and experienced. I know we have no grounds for insisting that Dr. Stevens do the biopsy, although I want to. Elena and I communicate all this and more through eye contact and hand squeezes.

We bring Liza into the room and tell her about this important test. Dr. Stevens tells Liza that she needs to lie on her stomach on the examining table and be as still as possible. He explains that Dr. Mueller will use a needle first to numb the skin above her tushy, touching the area on her left haunch so she understands where. The numbing medicine may sting for a minute, he adds, but it will make the test hurt much less. To keep her still, the grown-ups will hold her down. She already understands that the purpose of the test is to figure out the cause of her various pains and fevers over the last three weeks.

The doctors pull the examining table out from its usual position. As directed, we remove Liza's underpants. I give her a boost onto the table. Elena and I go behind the table and stand beside Liza to be out of the doctors' way. She lies facedown. Elena leans in by her head, holding our daughter's arms and shoulders. I lean across Liza's upper back. We realize that if she flails, it might botch the procedure, leading to repeated needles, more pain for her, more anxiety for everyone, and that perhaps the doctors would ask us to leave. So we intend to hold her firmly, white-knuckle firmly.

Liza remains quiet and poised, but I can see fear in her wide eyes. She is breathing faster. In soft voices, Elena and I assure her, "We are right here with you, Lizie. We'll help you through it."

Dr. Mueller prepares the equipment, specimen jars, and slides. Dr. Stevens guides us, adjusting our positions slightly, telling us where to stay. Two nurses come in to help. At Dr. Mueller's signal, they grab hold of Liza's legs. The doctor, announcing her actions to Liza and to us, injects a local anesthetic in the rear of Liza's left hip, over what I recall is named the iliac crest. Liza shrieks and cries. After a few minutes to allow the lidocaine to work, Dr. Mueller pushes a huge needle beneath the skin into Liza's hip. Liza screams, tenses, and tries to flinch her body away from the attacking metal, but we hold her down. Now I see why the additional nurses were needed. Elena starts counting with Liza, and I join in—at first "one Mississippi, two Mississippi..."—and then just the numbers themselves. Counting helps mark the passing seconds, helps Liza to hear us through her howls, to feel us with her. Counting slowly also makes each of us breathe more slowly, reducing our panic.

Dr. Mueller draws back a syringe full of deep red liquid.

"Is that it?" I ask.

"That is the bone marrow aspirate," Dr. Stevens explains. "Now we get the bone marrow biopsy, and then we are done." Dr. Mueller now grips the handle of a menacingly thick needle, more stick than needle, its center filled with a hollow metal plunger. A small woman, Dr. Mueller uses her entire body weight in the procedure, lifting onto her toes and leaning over Liza's hip as she drives the device in and twists. The extraction fails.

I stare at Dr. Stevens, and he understands my unspoken plea; he will make the next try. He snaps on a fresh pair of gloves, takes Dr. Mueller's needle and her place. Swifter and more certain, he rapidly bores into Liza's hip and then withdraws. This time the plunger holds the core of tissue. The procedure is over.

Liza is sobbing, and we cry with her. Elena and I stop counting and nestle around Liza, holding each other's hands and comforting her. For a few minutes, we take turns applying pressure where the stick has entered. A nurse checks that the bleeding has stopped and applies a bandage. Elena pulls up Liza's underwear, and Liza gingerly shifts her position. Leaning on us, she catches her breath and stops crying.

* * *

For four years running, in the early evening of Halloween, we have met with our neighborhood friends Penny and Bob and their kids to ransack their huge apartment building for candy. Now Liza wears her Simba costume from *The Lion King*, and Molly wears her policewoman costume, complete with helmet, handcuffs, and protective vest with prominent badge. I try to remember what characters Liza has inhabited on the three previous Halloweens. She was a fairy princess with wings and a magic wand last year, when she was three. Before that, was she Gumby, wearing that funny green mask? I can't recall what she was the year before, and I am fairly sure she was not costumed when she was only two weeks old. Will she live to celebrate other Halloweens in all the other costumes she can imagine? I push the thought away.

As we walk the six blocks down First Avenue just after dark, my beeper goes off. It is a shrill sound. From a street phone, I call Dr. Stevens.

"The bone marrow shows leukemia. Unmistakably, acute lymphocytic leukemia."

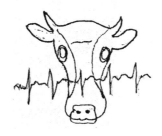

2—DAY ZERO
November 1994

The next day, we return early to Sinai's pediatric hematology-oncology clinic, and the nurse takes Liza's vital signs—her pulse, blood pressure, and weight. Before she can take blood as part of the check-in routine, I explain that Liza's blood was taken recently in the ER and that no treatment has yet begun, so I suspect this blood sample is not necessary. We want to spare Liza any unnecessary pain. From our own doctoring, Elena and I know how cavalierly blood tests are ordered for convenience. Surprised by my request, the nurse says that this is "simply routine," but she nonetheless agrees to hold off and check with the doctors.

The waiting room is overflowing with children of all ages, many of whom show the effects of chemotherapy: pale skin, bald scalp, skinny limbs. A few teenagers jut out from the furniture, all knees and elbows, more gangly and strange than ordinary strange-looking, gangly teenagers. They spill out from the chairs, fitting neither those for kids nor those for grown-ups. The hip-hop attire on the boys—baggy pants sliding down the hips to show a few inches of boxer shorts—is even more pronounced on their chemotherapy-ravaged bodies. Some are unaccompanied, a show of independence that seems odd to see in the young, when Elena and I feel so protective. Several of the teenagers appear robust, despite their cancer, and this is heartening to see. Most of the parents sag with weariness. This crowd frightens me.

Doctors come to the waiting area and greet their patients one by one. Tentatively, Liza goes over to a play kitchenette, checks out the various utensils, cookware, and plastic pears, oranges, waffles at hand, then returns to reclaim her seat with us. Dr. Stevens appears and says, "Hi, Liza."

She mumbles, "Hi."

He adds, "I need to talk with your mom and dad for a little while." He escorts us down the same hall we walked yesterday, and when we pass the room where Liza's biopsy was done, I hear her shrieks. I flinch and then steel myself.

In today's larger examining room, the medical staff is seated in a circle of chairs with small side desktops. Dr. Stevens introduces the team. There's Dr. Mueller, of course, the fellow, his junior colleague, along with a social worker and two nurse practitioners, one of whom, Lucy, helped hold Liza down yesterday and the other I recognize as the one wearing the doggy costume yesterday.

Also present are two medical students who are not named. One sits on a table directly across from us, slightly behind Dr. Stevens. I glare at her, angry that medical students are invited now to sit in on our lives. I don't want to be here, but if I have to be here, I want to find grounds for demanding that the students be ousted. But this young woman gives no such cause. She is attentive, involved, respectful, clearly moved, and yet composed. I envy her "outsideness." It's something I'm familiar with myself, actually, from my training in and later practice of psychiatry—the safe position of observer and helper, imbued with concern, curiosity, confidence, and imagined invincibility. For a moment, I escape by wondering how the experience appears through her eyes. Quickly, I assail myself with silent questions: *Is this real? Is this really happening? Is there any escaping?*

I look at these people, needing them to give us their best, aware that when this meeting ends, they will go to other meetings and other duties, while we will be powerless to move away. Their faces are comforting in their steadiness, conveying open hearts and actively working minds, but then I glance at the male medical student in the corner, the only one in the room standing. As he leans against the counter, he keeps shifting his position restlessly, eyes on the floor.

Maybe he's just tired from being on call, but I don't think that's it. He seems detached and bored, wishing he weren't here.

Elena and I sit beside each other, holding hands. Our isolation cannot be remedied. On this day, Tuesday morning, November 1, in this cramped room full of strangers, I realize that our lives have been changed forever. These people we are looking at, and who are looking at us, will get to know us very well.

Dr. Stevens begins the meeting. "We call this the 'Day Zero talk.' Acute lymphocytic leukemia, ALL, is the most common childhood cancer. Conventional treatment lasts two full years, twenty-four months, beginning today. Tests of Liza's bone marrow reveal that her kind of leukemic cells resemble precursors of B lymphocytes. Pre-B cell leukemia is the most successfully treated. The cure rate is high, now greater than 80 percent. Research over the past two decades has brought tremendous gains. Liza has no known high-risk factors. She is an otherwise healthy girl in an age range most successfully treated."

As Dr. Stevens speaks, we are given handouts, information about all of the treatment medicines. A sample month-to-a-page calendar for a "standard-risk" patient such as Liza shows when she needs to come to the clinic or be admitted for treatment, when she will need bone marrow biopsies, spinal taps, when different medicines start and stop. The team seems well organized, but soon Elena and I are holding a jumble of papers. I feel sensitive to the smallest flaw, the page with blurry print or with words cut off in the photocopying, as if this sloppiness could be deadly. Outweighing such distractions are Dr. Stevens's experience, his steady voice, and patient eyes. I try to concentrate on that.

He simplifies for us all the information we are receiving. "Treatment consists of three stages: Induction comes first, then consolidation." As soon as I hear the name of the third stage, it escapes me. Maintenance? Recovery? Blossoming? Renewal? Making Everything All Better? No matter—I'll have time to find out what it's called later.

Lucy, the dark-haired, dark-eyed nurse practitioner, is a woman of high energy and rapid speech. She explains the plan for surgically placing a central line in Liza, formally called a "Broviac catheter." The Broviac tube is inserted under the skin of the chest into a large vein, with the tip resting near the heart; when not in use, its dangling end, above the skin's surface, is capped, taped, and pinned to the patient's clothing. The Broviac catheter helps both the patient and the medical team by making it painless and easy to administer medicine and obtain blood samples through just one stable channel, instead of an endless barrage of needle pricks.

Lucy tells us that the simple operation will be scheduled for tomorrow morning or, at the latest, the day after. She speaks generally about the need to maintain the catheter, but she understands we cannot absorb the information at the moment and will discuss specifics in the days ahead. "Since you are both doctors, I'm sure taking care of the catheter will be easy for you," she says. I hope she's not wrong in expecting us to be more detached, more competent, and less anxious than we are. We could sneeze and contaminate the IV as easily as any other parent. She laughs when I mention the lethality of my sneezes and reassures us that she will teach us all we need to know and will not expect us to do any more than we're comfortable doing.

During much of the conference, Elena and I cry intermittently. It is a contained and quiet crying, sometimes together, sometimes in turn. Often one of us is calmed and strengthened by leaning on the other; sometimes the tears of one set the other to crying anew. The medical staff wait respectfully. They give us the time we need, generous in an hour that feels timeless, except for moments when we experience Liza's absence, so far away down the hall. I wonder what she is feeling and thinking, waiting for us.

Dr. Stevens responds to our many questions, even the impossible ones: Why do people get leukemia? Why did Liza get leukemia? Why this child, not her sister, why not some other child, why not one of us? Is the place we live in dangerous, full of some invisible toxin? Elena and I break into sobs together when Dr. Stevens says, "You did nothing wrong. You did not cause the illness." Our tears burn, and we clutch each other for a few moments. He has addressed a fear we held more deeply than we knew.

"And if the treatment doesn't work?" I ask.

"There are options," he replies vaguely. He notes the possibility of more powerful chemotherapy given to high-risk patients, or bone marrow transplant, a treatment basically foreign to us. He is clearly not inclined to say more about this now.

Toward the end of the meeting, Dr. Stevens says, "You will need to decide whether to participate in Mount Sinai's ongoing leukemia study." The largest handout we've been given describes the study and includes a multipage consent form. I can scarcely retain what he's telling us about the research—I can find the details in the handout later—but I gather that several variables are being studied: medicines or doses different than the current default treatment. Dr. Stevens assures us that even if we choose the conventional treatment for Liza and abstain from the research study, she will receive the same level of excellent medical care and commitment. In the research study, of the six medications ordinarily used in treatment, three are given in altered form or dosage because there is reason to believe that each alteration may promote an improved outcome. The total time course of the treatment protocol is the same—two years either way. We can agree to participate in one, two, or three "arms" of the experiment, or in none.

"When do we need to decide?"

"In the next hour." The feeling that time had been suspended vanishes. Dr. Stevens adjourns the meeting so Elena and I can weigh the research question and decide.

I call a few of the pediatricians we know best—old friends, Elena's uncle, doctors I trained with—and put them on the spot. "If you were in my place, if this was your daughter, what would you do?" But I also use them to hear myself articulate and organize the thoughts that Elena and I quickly produced: *Risk of participation: possible worse side effects. Benefit of participation: possible more effective treatment.* A research study undergoes intense scrutiny before it is approved, and only with strong grounds to hope for greater efficacy would new treatment options reach clinical trials, which is what Liza would be involved in. *The benefit of nonparticipation: confidence in a high rate of cure under circumstances tried and true, involving a minimum of surprises. The risk of nonparticipation: complex.* If Liza is not cured, we might feel that we did not try every treatment mode available. For a moment, I let myself think the unbearable—Liza could die from this illness—before returning to the decision we have to make.

I gesture to Elena: *Join me.* We decide to participate in the study and sign the consent. Dr. Stevens takes the form and explains that now we are going to be "randomized." We already feel randomized enough. Now a computer will conduct a lottery to determine the forms and dosages of the medicines Liza will receive.

An hour after we agree to participate, we learn the result of randomization. Liza will receive the experimental form of medicine in all three arms of the study. How strange—after sweating out whether to participate, we might just as easily have been put into the control group for all three arms and received the conventional treatment. We feel fortunate to be getting the most aggressive treatments, apparently the very best chance for cure. Quietly, however, we also acknowledge to each other that we are scared. More scared than we have ever been in our lives.

Reflections in the Rearview Mirror

Who Attends?

I know I reacted strongly to the medical students being at the meeting. Their presence underscored the helplessness I was feeling. On reflection, I sympathize with the two of them, neither properly introduced, neither given a proper seat. If I sensed correctly that the male didn't want to be there, perhaps he had good reasons—kindhearted reasons, even. Maybe the whole experience disturbed him. Maybe he felt he shouldn't be a spectator to something of such personal importance to us.

If I had a magic wand, I would've framed the meeting differently—it's a framework in which Elena and I would've been less uncomfortable, along with the students. Dr. Stevens would've taken the leadership initiative of speaking to the students in advance: "We are about to have a meeting that will likely be very emotionally intense for the parents, but I am including you on purpose," he could have said. "No matter what branch of medicine you go into, you will probably have to face breaking bad news to people. So don't feel that you are being included by accident or thoughtlessly. We can debrief afterward." They would have been seated at desks like everyone else, introduced by name like everyone else.

Then, after the introductions, I'd have Dr. Stevens make a similar statement to us. "We include medical students purposely. This kind of meeting will be invaluable to them for the rest of their careers." Had he introduced them and said something of the sort to us, I believe I would have been more at peace with their presence and they, in turn, would have been able to engage fully. I have the sense that the female student immersed herself despite the disadvantages.

Imagine that these two students represent two parts of one person. I think we all have the capacity to be empathically present and connected or, if activated, to disengage. I know I do. So many factors contribute to one's ability to engage or not: how many hours of sleep they've had, their tolerance for emotionality and vulnerability, their awareness of their level of stress or of being triggered by a difficult conversation. All of these things contribute to a person's mindful ability to settle themselves and reengage when called for. That level of cognizance takes dedication from every helper on the team, on an individual basis. Within a group, leadership has a huge impact, and the leadership effort I call for in my reimagined framework would not have been a huge one.

But there's something else I would change about that day. Someone is missing from the Day Zero talk, I realized years later, after having had so many more momentous conversations with our team of helpers, so many discussions about relapse, about facing unexpected complications, about Liza being terminal. Later, we worked with doctors specializing in palliative care within the hospital setting, and finally, we worked with a hospice. There is a place for hospice as a specific organized framework for care at the end of life, but the attitude embodied by hospice, which is also carried by the palliative care team, should not be separated from ongoing care.

So, when I wield my magic wand again, a palliative care specialist would have been at the Day Zero meeting. This specialist would have articulated something like, "We understand that the treatment ahead will be grueling at times, but we are prepared to offer support as needed throughout, no matter how smooth or bumpy the road. We view Liza's comfort as key to her and your entire family's morale. So we will be alert to any impediments to her comfort—pain, itching, fatigue, worry."

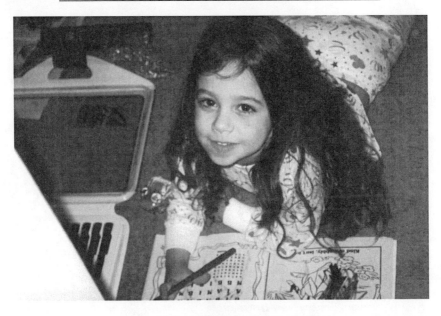

Liza with workbook, February 1994.

It would be nice if every member of every oncology team every-where reflected this point of view. If that were the case, there mightn't be a need for palliative care teams at all. But we aren't there yet. Per-haps we'll get there in a couple generations' time, but for now, we need specialists to lead us in prioritizing the comfort of the patient. I believe this should be as important at the beginning of the medical journey as it is at the end. If we'd met our palliative care specialist on November 1, 1994, we'd have known where to turn later, when Liza started encountering extreme pain. Our specialist would have inter-vened swiftly, advocating effectively for better pain control, so that I wouldn't have needed to hound the staff at the nursing station. Which I did. Repeatedly. To the exasperation of all.

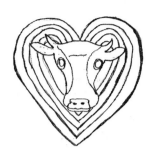

3—INDUCTION

November 1994

Knowing Liza will spend the next month in the hospital, Elena and I quickly reorganize our lives so that we can take turns staying with her at night. Whichever one of us wakes at the hospital will stay on for part of the morning. It is in those early-morning hours that doctors come on rounds, and it will be an important opportunity to ask questions. Some days, Elena and I pass the baton to each other directly. Other days, Cleveth, our beautiful-hearted Jamaican babysitter, will come to the hospital for a spell in the late morning and stay into the afternoon, until the other parent arrives. Cleveth has been with us since Molly was a few weeks old, and both girls are very close to her.

"Can you guys please be quiet?" Liza asks when she is weary. If peppy, she wants to play cards or have a story. When we are both at the hospital, Liza wants us to attend to *her*, not for us to catch up with each other or go for a hospital stroll without her. Liza has to handle both the reunion with the parent who is staying and the imminent departure of the parent who is leaving. While one stays, the other parent goes to work and then home to have one-on-one time with Molly.

I suggest to Elena that we keep a notebook in Liza's night table, and she agrees. Elena finds a notebook with a blue and purple plaid cover, perfect because they are Liza's favorite colors. It becomes our

19

own private medical chart and journal. Elena and I note our observations and concerns, questions we want to ask the doctors, lab results of importance, doctors who have come by. We write not only the date, but also the number of the day. If today is Day Zero, tomorrow is Day 1. We write down Liza's comments and questions, her responses to all the intrusions of illness, her quirky phrases, things we'd share if we were together, like:

> Day 3: Tummy hurting. Urine turned red from medicine.
> Day 4: Molly's first visit, Liza was cheerful for that but afterward apathetic.
> Day 6: Liza: "I had a dream of being outside a house where some fighting is going on inside. And in another dream, I saw two birthday cakes like the ones at Erica's birthday, one all white, one with pink and purple icing."
> Day 9: Liza: "I wish I did not have such a big sickness, but just a little cough for a day or two. I want to be outside and feel the wind and see the sun. I want to go home. Having to stay in the hospital makes me cranky!"

Molly and Liza are effectively separated from each other from Sunday evening to the next weekend. Elena and I have less time together than ever before. Sweeping aside our routines, I see how much I count on Elena for support and everyday companionship. We all speak by phone every night, Liza and one parent taking turns on the hospital room phone, and Molly and the home parent exchanging the blue phone with the long, coiled cord in our bedroom. More important than any news updates, we hear one another's voices and say good night.

We understand that within one to two weeks of the start of her treatment, Liza's hair will fall out. We prepare her. "Lizie, the medicine you are getting is going to kill the sick white blood cells, but it also kills other cells in the body, including the cells that make your hair, and your hair is going to fall out. The good news is that it will tell us that the medicine is working. And when the medicine is finished, your hair will grow back." But more powerful than our words is Liza's quiet observation of other children without hair in the clinic and on the hospital ward. Her own hair is long, wavy, curly at the bottom. It rolls onto her shoulders, a beautiful golden brown, lighter than anyone else's in the family, almost blond in spots. In contrast, her olive skin is the darkest complexion in the family. Her round face of toddler years is giving way to more sculpted, angular cheeks. Her large, soulful hazel eyes give her a slightly exotic look. Slim and strong, she is a fast runner. In recent weeks, playing catch in the park, Liza would clutch the football tenaciously and, with shoulders squared, dash in random circles and figure eights after catching a toss.

When the fourteenth day passes without her hair changing visibly, Elena and I are surprised, confused. I even fantasize that Liza has received a waiver: Her beautiful hair has communicated covertly with the medicines and reached a unique accord. Might the medicines spare Liza their notorious ill effects? Might she have the easiest course of leukemia treatment ever known? In this way, Nature could apologize for its preposterous mistake.

A few days later, though, it starts to happen. As Liza and Elena prepare to settle in for the evening, Elena brushes her hair. They both notice that the hairbrush is filling up, and even though we all expected it, nothing blunts the shock. Still, Liza instructs, "Keep brushing." The brush collects ever more hair, at first loose strands and tendrils, but then tufts and clumps. Liza sobs into her mother's chest. "I don't want to lose my hair."

"I know, sweetheart," Elena says. "It will take some getting used to. But you'll be okay with it. You are wonderful and beautiful with or without hair. And remember: This means the medicine is working to kill the sick white blood cells. Your hair will grow back and stay. But you should feel proud and good about yourself no matter what happens to your hair."

Liza cries herself to sleep.

The next day, she exuberantly tells Molly and Nanny and me all about losing her hair. Using Elena's script, she declares, "I'm going to get used to it no matter what! And it means that the medicines are working to kill the sick white blood cells." Nevertheless, Liza feels like her scalp is on fire, burning with the weight of her dead hair. She wants the feeling to stop. Thirty-six hours after the hair loss started, she asks us, "Daddy, Mommy, please just cut off my hair." We do. Baldness radically alters Liza's appearance, revealing a new beauty.

＊　＊　＊

From the outset, Liza has been given huge doses of an intravenous steroid. This medication makes her moody—at times irritable, at times funny—and voraciously hungry. Hunger is a problem on days before a procedure, when she is not allowed to eat or drink—NPO (nothing by mouth), as the sign on her door shouts. Liza's understanding of the medical reasons for this deprivation does little to help. She cries—ravenous, angry, and helpless. Elena and I feel trapped even as we try everything we can think of to distract her. Some nights, to minimize her torment the next morning, we keep her up past midnight and then let her sleep late.

Liza begins to pick at her fingernails and toenails. Sometimes she picks willfully, but often the picking appears to be mindless. The steroids probably cause it, we know. Should we leave her alone? Liza declares, "These are *my* fingers and toes, not yours!"

"But your body is also ours to care for and protect," I reply.

Because we are forced to limit Liza in many things, we want to allow her freedom where we can. But seeing her pull back her nails is excruciating to witness, more so for me than Elena. I try to model my wife's patience. But when Liza hurts herself, when she bleeds, she risks infection. It's clear we have to break her of this habit, but it's hard to enforce. She resists being told what to do. Red-faced, she fumes, "Leave me alone!" Later, contrite, she promises to try to stop, but then she starts again distractedly, picking the cuticles and probing the corners of her nails, bending them back. Sometimes, angry and defiant, she just wants to pick for satisfaction, even if it means pain. When we interfere, she screams. We have to remind ourselves over and over that Liza isn't herself right now, made crazy by the steroids, so that we don't scream back or collapse in anguish.

Band-Aids! It dawns on me that if I can offer Band-Aids that appeal to her, it might stem the picking. Elena and I hunt in every pharmacy we pass, collecting varieties that Liza will enjoy, especially ones with designs from *Beauty and the Beast, The Little Mermaid,* and *101 Dalmatians.* She agrees to try them to cover her nails, and soon putting them on becomes an obsessional task for her, for us all. As she playfully decorates her hands and feet, she permits me to act as her manicurist. I smooth a rough or broken nail, preparing the fingers for wrapping. Liza and I work hard to get each bandage oriented correctly, sticking snugly but not too tightly. At her direction, I use the scissors on my pocketknife to shorten the ends of the Band-Aid or to cut one into two narrower strips, especially for her pinkies and baby toes. Liza enjoys this innovation and requests, "Will you make some of those smaller ones for Mommy to use tomorrow?" Working with Liza's nails becomes a zany delight, a version of playing beauty shop. But when she loses her sense of humor (or we ours), Liza can become insanely meticulous and impossible to satisfy.

"This one is too loose. See, I can pull it right off. No! Now it's too tight!"

"Enough, Liza!" I blurt. Elena and I each get mad at her—but fortunately, not too often.

* * *

AIR IN LINE ... AIR IN LINE ... AIR IN LINE. The red block letters scroll across the screen of the high-tech infusion pump, the vehicle for delivering many of Liza's medications and transfusions. Accompanying the alarming words, the machine emits piercing beeps as if a truck is backing up into our hospital room, and it seems to happen often. When we buzz the nursing station, a voice sounding somewhat irritated responds through the wall intercom, "May I help you?" Sometimes, before we even answer, the voice registers the beeping and says curtly, "I'll send your nurse in to fix the IV."

Elena and I notice that the nurses almost always go by their first names with us, whereas the doctors use their surnames. Is this because the doctors hold authority and use intellect to strategize, assess, and oversee, with hearts more armored, while the nurses attend in a more basic way to Liza's comfort, her bodily needs? Drs. Stevens and Mueller continue as our principal team of attending physician and fellow. As we get to know them better, and they us, they refer to each other by first name, and in an organic way, we shift to calling them by their first names as well. As doctors, Elena and I know about hospital hierarchy, but as the parents of a patient, we learn it in a new way. Any of four other attendings may cover for Dr. Stevens. Any of four other fellows may rotate in for Dr. Mueller. A whirl of residents and interns in general pediatrics run the day-to-day business of the floor. We use our bedside notebook to keep track of the cast of characters, their names and roles. When we can slow them down for just a half measure and see them as named individuals, it seems that our interactions improve. They, in turn, seem more likely to see us as people too.

Liza is comforted to be accompanied by her beloved beanbag cow, her "cowie," in the hospital—even for every X-ray, every test— while her other cherished stuffed animals remain safely at home. Noticing this attachment leads our friends and relatives to search for any kind of bovine they can find, and Liza's collection grows. One cow sits upright, displaying a small red heart on its belly emblazoned with SQUEEZE ME, which produces a slow, deep low. This cow serves as a litmus test for people visiting her bedside. Upon seeing it, some people just snatch it up and squeeze—folks who feel entitled to grab what interests them, like the doctors who try to examine Liza regardless of her readiness or willingness to be inspected, tapped, prodded, or poked. Such behavior toward her red-hearted cow incenses Liza. Depending on her mood, she either becomes stony or shouts, "Put down my cow right now!" But when someone asks first, requests permission to hold and squeeze it, Liza almost always agrees, eagerly watching for their surprised reaction. When someone familiar comes, she might hide the cow behind her back and squeeze it secretly, startling the visitor with a mysterious "Moo."

Of all the physicians, one intern stands out for treating Liza's cows and Liza herself respectfully. Dr. Fein is a petite woman with pale skin, curly dark hair, and, behind glasses, dark eyes that are filled with intelligence, kindness, and, perhaps, some anxiety. Her first rotation on the fifth floor began right before Liza's admission, and she cares for Liza whenever she's on duty. Despite the harried schedule of internship, Dr. Fein lingers when she can, and she tries hard to get to know Liza. She is peppily efficient, good-humored, intuitive, and persistent. Even though Liza becomes angry when Dr. Fein disturbs her for blood samples or to examine her, the intern keeps trying to reach her. She sees Liza as a smart, sensitive four-year-old and speaks to her plainly, neither as a baby nor as an older kid. When Liza fusses, she asks her to explain her objections. Sometimes Dr. Fein backs off, only to try to engage Liza again soon. Before long, she succeeds. She actually tells us her first name—Carolyn. To us, she seems startlingly young.

One afternoon, Carolyn comes into the room and sees that Liza is sleeping. She quietly tells Elena and me, "I understand what you guys are going through—why you are so vigilant. My parents were exactly the same way. I had cancer as a child, and seeing you reminds me of them. They were very involved and protective." Though she speaks dispassionately, her words stir us deeply. Trusting our judgment, she allows us to tell her story to Liza, if we wish. When we do, Liza listens and makes little comment, but she seems pleased. Elena and I greatly appreciate Carolyn's openness, combined with her intelligent and sympathetic care. To us, she embodies a statistic come to life, the possibility of cure. Not only has she survived her own early encounter with cancer and the rigors of medical training, but she has survived with her humanity intact. Meeting her is a potent boon, and I realize that I've been carrying around an underground pool of fear that Liza may not survive ... and even if she does, that she may be severely scarred from the experience.

Overall, Liza's induction—the initial course of treatment aiming to remove all clinically detectable cancer—goes well. She needs only a few transfusions of red blood cells, and we'd been warned she might have needed many more. She encounters only one mild bout of pneumonia, which responds quickly to treatment, and we'd also been warned that infections could be a serious, repeated problem. Her chemotherapy constipates her, and she is given laxatives. At first, too strong, they cause crampy diarrhea, but through trial and error, the right dose is established. Liza cooperates with taking a few dozen medicines daily. If they are in tablet form, we grind them up and hide them creatively—in juice, ice cream, yogurt, chocolate syrup. When she has nausea, stomachaches, or diffuse pain, she is given additional medicine. We are on a merry-go-round of anti-leukemia drugs, drugs to offset the side effects of the anti-leukemia drugs, and other drugs to offset those.

Mostly, Liza maintains good cheer. In her hospital room, she engages in private make-believe play, especially at bedtime. I overhear bits and pieces of her whispery, affectionate voice animating her special possessions, including, always, her beanbag cowie, a small stuffed Curious George, and, interestingly enough, a blue bandana. "Yes, exactly!" one of these declares to another, who understands perfectly.

At the beginning of our fourth week in the hospital, with discharge in sight, Liza says to Elena, "I'm much bigger now. It's almost like I'm almost five, really, because I got so much bigger in this hospital being here so long. I'm working on helping to get me all better. I think once you get rid of this sickness, it never comes back. You never get it again." We see no reason to tamper with this belief, which stems from last year, when she and Molly had chicken pox.

Liza occasionally asks questions, particularly about each new medicine, but mostly she demonstrates her complete faith in our judgment. We anticipate her potential bafflement, and whenever we can, we offer her information about what to expect. Talking about the treatment calms us all and draws us closer. When she had pneumonia, for example, we gave Liza advance notice about the X-rays and the nebulizer treatments. Whenever new medicines are ordered and whenever food will be restricted or procedures are to be performed, Elena and I decide together what to tell Liza and when. She doesn't need preparation for trivial matters, but for her, little is trivial. On the other hand, giving her too much information too soon can provoke anxiety rather than comfort her.

A similar process evolves with Molly. As Liza's appearance changes, Molly needs a chance to voice her observations and concerns and to ask questions. She notes astutely, "Liza's face is different, and so is her voice. Her cheeks are puffier, and her voice is...." Molly's forehead furrows as she searches for the right word.

"Huskier?" I offer. She nods. "That's from one of the medicines."

"Which medicine?"

"The steroid. And when the steroid is going up or down, when she is taking more or less, she gets especially moody, and it can be really tough not to anger her. So we'll let you know if that's going on before you visit this weekend."

A flurry of arrangements precede our discharge, including lessons in taking care of the Broviac catheter. We get Liza's medications from the hospital pharmacy and write a schedule for giving them. We are to be released on a Wednesday, the day before Thanksgiving. I ask Dot, a friend who is a skilled seamstress, to make some hats for Liza, should Liza want to cover her head. Dot quickly provides me with seven hats and caps that I bring to the hospital and show Liza.

To complete her hospital departure outfit, Liza selects her favorite, a teal velour number with a large, lacy purple flower and purple feathers on the front brim—very stylish indeed for her first time dressed in anything but pajamas in almost a month.

We walk out of the room we are glad to vacate and go to the nursing station where we first stood almost a month earlier. We say goodbye to the nurses and the doctors who are there. I carry Liza on my shoulders. We feel triumphant to have weathered so much so well and to be released almost a week ahead of the original forecast. Liza's face is rounder from the steroids, her skin paler, and she is weak. But she beams as we make our getaway.

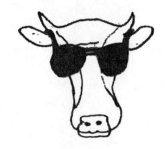

4—A Bumpy Road
November–December 1994

We are glad to be home for Thanksgiving, the only meaningful holiday for our family. Eating may be the closest thing we have to a religion, and we embrace the ideal of a grateful heart along with a full belly. Accompanying our relief and gladness is a sense of letdown as we get used to being home. Elena and I have to find ways to share the new responsibilities that have been added to our old ones. When we took turns at the hospital, our duties were unmistakable. But now that we're all home, nothing divides "on duty" from "off." We muddle toward new patterns. I am livid at the fact of leukemia, but I don't know how to argue with it. So I gripe and bicker with Elena instead, and she returns the favor.

"Lainie, where did you put the clicker?"

"You always blame me, when I wasn't using the TV at all."

"Did you throw out the leftover soup?"

"I smelled it, and it had gone bad."

"That's ridiculous! I just had some this afternoon."

"Then those must have been your dishes that were left in the sink."

These petty bothers are familiar, but now they carry all of our disgust with illness, all of our fear of not knowing where it will lead.

While we bounce down this emotional stairway, the girls go

through similar struggles once they determine that life is secure enough to permit everyday sibling squabbles.

Liza seems feisty enough for Molly to quarrel with safely. "I want to use the markers, Molly."

"You're just saying that because you see me starting to use them."

"I like sitting in this spot on the couch, and you got to sit here whenever you wanted when I was in the hospital."

"That's not fair, Lizie. We have to share it. You can sit there now, but I get to have a turn too."

While it is irritating to see the girls struggle, it is also reassuring—and challenging. When I see Liza trying to make Molly feel guilty, I step in. "Lize, it's not Molly's fault that you got sick. She's worried about you and missed you, and you guys need to figure out how to share stuff just like you used to."

The task of helping them adjust returns Elena and me to our sense of working as a team. I tell her what happened and ask, "Do you think I was right to butt in and support Molly there?"

"Usually, you're the one who suggests that I step in too soon," Elena says. "So if you felt the need to step in, it was probably a good idea, and it sounds like it was. I hope you can give me the same benefit of the doubt when I do it."

"I hope I can too." We chuckle. "It's easy to see the wisdom of letting them work it out themselves when *you're* the one stepping in!"

"Butting in, you mean," she says. At the moment, we can laugh when we think we're getting it right, but it's just as easy to get uptight and defensive. I recognize those moments when Elena steps away abruptly, steaming when I suggest she back off. And I have my own sulky way of withdrawing when stung by her criticism.

We also weave medical matters into our new daily routine. With vigilant attention to sterile technique, we take turns caring for the Broviac catheter—flushing the line and changing the caps. When it comes to changing the dressing and cleaning the site where the catheter emerges from Liza's skin, I am tense, afraid of making missteps and causing infection, afraid of hurting Liza by being too rough or damaging the catheter's placement. Struggling to contain my discomfort but intent on carrying out the multistep procedure carefully, correctly, and quickly, I resist the urge to bow out from changing her dressings altogether. To steady and calm myself, I hum one of Liza's favorite lullabies while I fret, and Liza relaxes, occasionally humming along for a bit. Often by the time I finish, she has fallen asleep. Her breathing is characteristically heavy and congested, not quite a snore, a trademark since babyhood.

Her trust here moves me, and I remind myself of it during difficult moments when she verbally, and at times physically, pushes me away. "No, I want Mommy!" Sometimes she clings to Elena for days at a time. I know I should be big enough to not let this bother me, but at times I feel hurt and sag. *What did I do wrong?* I wonder. I tell myself that it is temporary; I rest and bounce back. If I need to check with Elena, she reassures me. I understand Liza's need to pull Elena close. More difficult than with any toy or chair, she is relearning to share her mommy with Molly.

*　*　*

A couple of days after getting home, Lisa Mueller phones in the late afternoon and tells us that the marrow appears "completely normal." We are elated to hear the results of what Liza calls the "bow 'n' arrow test." It means Liza has successfully completed the induction phase: Her leukemia is "in remission."

In remission. We embrace the good news, but a few days later, we realize that we don't know exactly what the term means. Did I skip that class in medical school or doze through it? Does it mean that the leukemia is all gone? If all gone, the coming twenty-three months of treatment we have been told to plan on would be unnecessary. It must mean *almost* all gone. Come to think of it, one of the doctors mentioned a definition—a figure, a large number, an exponent, ten-to-the-something power of leukemic cells or, rather, less-than-ten-to-the-something power ... less than that number of leukemic cells remaining. I can ask the doctor to tell me the number again, and I can write it in our medical notebook. I can know that number. But why?

I do understand that for treatment to be effective, it must eliminate the vast majority of sick cells, so that one day Liza's own defenses can take over. The coming chemotherapy aims to kill that large number of remaining leukemic cells. I try out various metaphors to make sense of the quandary of medical language. Maybe Liza's bone marrow is like a garden overgrown with weeds. First, we pull out the visible ones, but afterward, and for a time, formerly hidden weeds will appear. We will have to be vigilant for a long time if we are to have any chance of saving the garden from the weeds taking over again. Some healthy flowers and shrubs may be lost in the effort. Or perhaps Liza's body is like a country overtaken by an invading enemy. First, and with relative ease, we battle the visible battalions of the enemy. But then, though in apparent retreat, the enemy scatters and resorts to guerrilla warfare, infiltrating the tangled vegetation. This requires a major, sustained effort to search out and destroy the enemy forces one by one. They are unlikely to ever surrender.

❊   ❊   ❊

Elena and I walk a fine line navigating between, on the one side, our urge to protect Liza at all costs and avoid any risk of exposing her to danger and, on the other, our wish that she live each day fully. Whenever she feels well enough, we encourage her to explore the world. We make family outings to the Central Park Zoo, to the nearby open-air market, and to St. Catherine's Park, what we call "the market park." In the days that follow, we take Liza to lunch, to dinner, and to Hanukkah celebrations. She enjoys them with gusto. After almost a month in the hospital, she grasps that these ordinary experiences are not to be taken for granted. Strikingly, she shows no concern for her altered appearance—bald head, paler skin except for rounder and redder cheeks, eyebrows and lashes that stand out beautifully, fuller torso but with slightly skinnier arms and legs, huskier voice, posture a trace less erect. If it is warm enough when we go out, she often opts to wear no hat. If she does wear a hat, she removes it unselfconsciously when she feels like it. Elena and I relish her resilience, her confident demeanor, and her thoughtful and humorously delivered opinions. But we remain alert, listening closely for any sneeze, any cough.

❊   ❊   ❊

Our home-based time is interrupted by short stays in the hospital for planned overnight infusions of chemo. Unplanned short stays for antibiotics are required for low-grade fevers. Through it all, Liza discovers and declares her strength in a variety of ways. "Look, I can snap my fingers! I can push open my room door. I can get the ice without spilling any. I can unplug my IV and walk down the hall with my IV pole!" After rubbing her eye, she finds a stray eyelash on her fingertip; with eyes closed, she wishes on her eyelash "for everyone to never get sick," and then she opens her eyes and blows the eyelash away. She tells us that she likes knowing about her illness and appreciates the way we answer her questions. "I know all about my sickness and medicines because you and Mommy tell me, and I don't forget because, if I understand, then I don't worry about what is happening."

*   *   *

After six weeks home, one evening after work when I approach the dining room, Elena tells me quickly and privately that Liza, who is sitting at the dinner table, is feeling lousy. I greet Liza and feel her head; it is not warm, but hot. We take her temperature: 103. Even before we reach the doctor on call, we know what we must do.

Reflections in the Rearview Mirror

How Is It Possible?

Not long after my dad died, Elena and I began thinking about having a second child, perhaps partly informed by wanting to move forward from my father's loss. But I worried that I wouldn't be able to love another child as much as I loved Molly.

"How will it be possible to love a new baby as much?" I asked my mom.

She simply smiled and shook her head. "You don't need to worry. You'll find out. It'll be okay."

She seemed tuned in to the way the species is programmed. As she predicted, in time I did find out. When Liza was born, I discovered that there was something about parental love, maybe love in general, that defied the concrete idea I'd had, that there was a finite amount of it, like a certain number of gallons. It occurred to me that maybe love is like a reservoir, even as it keeps emptying, it keeps filling. Or maybe there's no reservoir at all. Maybe love is limitless. And if grief is the cost of love, as psychiatrist Colin Murray Parkes phrases it, maybe the capacity for grief is just as limitless.

* * *

"Do you have kids?" *Meeting someone new, I often anticipate the question, sense it coming like a tennis rally, knowing where the next shot will land.*

"Yes."

"How many?" *The obvious next shot usually, but not always, follows.*

"We have three."

Not two.

Sometimes the rally stops there. Sometimes I stop it, by looking away or taking control of the direction of the back-and-forth with another question. But if I don't evade, if the rally continues:

"How old?"

* * *

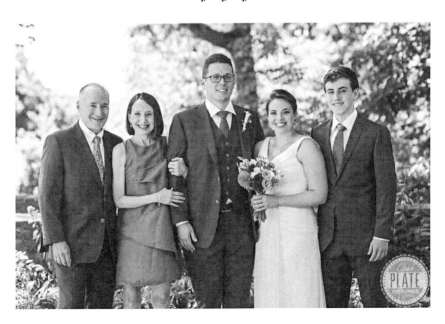

Molly and Jason marry, September 2016.

Our daughter Molly is thirty-one years old now, married, living half an hour away. Liza, who would have been twenty-eight, died twenty-three years ago. Our twenty-one-year-old son, Solomon, is in college. Although Liza died, she is still our child. She still counts.

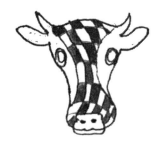

5—COMPLICATIONS
January–March 1995

A t the hospital, culture results show that a common fungus is growing in one of Liza's blood specimens. With their defenses intact, most people never succumb to fungal infections, but with Liza's defenses suppressed by chemotherapy, she is vulnerable to such opportunists. She must be in a single room.

Our general pediatrician, Dr. Raucher, who happens to be an infectious disease specialist, answers the many questions we have. Though he does not participate directly in Liza's care, he stops by her hospital room every day. Frequently, if she is awake when he comes by, she simply rejects his efforts to engage her by sullenly refusing to respond to him. But Elena and I are glad that we are on his daily radar, and we welcome the sight of his large frame, his long stride, his thoroughly predictable manner: friendly, patient, optimistic, grounded, sober. Whenever something is inconclusive or uncertain, he speaks to us frankly—he is our back channel to the medical chart and to the decision-making of the doctors in charge. We catch him on his early-morning rounds, and we speak in the hall while Liza sleeps. Whether it is his knowledge of us or of people in general, he understands Elena's and my tendency to blame ourselves. He assures us that this infection is not the result of our faulty care of Liza. We feel greatly relieved by his certainty, his clear synthesis. But at the same time, it is painful to realize we now face a significant hurdle.

Because fungal infections can be life-threatening and are almost impossible to eliminate with an indwelling catheter, the Broviac must be removed immediately. A surgery fellow arrives. Snickering at our worried questions, he declares, "I can whip it out anytime, right here on the ward in Liza's room." On receiving the go-ahead from the hematology-oncology team, he dons mask and sterile gloves and uncovers Liza's upper body. He removes the dressing, snips a stitch, and pulls the three-foot-long catheter from Liza's chest swiftly, steadily. Elena comforts her and applies pressure to a gauze pad until a nurse checks the site and tapes on a fresh bandage.

Without the Broviac, Liza frequently suffers needles for blood collections, and although she does not scream or cry, we can see that they hurt. Whenever one IV stops working, a new one is inserted. Liza tries to keep each new IV site—whether it be in hand, arm, or foot—completely still, so it will last and more needle sticks can be avoided.

The drug for treating Liza's fungal infection, amphotericin, can be wicked, and Liza reacts severely to a test dose with fever and itching. To minimize the side effects, she is premedicated with steroids and other medications, including an antihistamine to prevent fever, itching, and hives, before starting the six-hour infusion of amphotericin. The antihistamine knocks her out; when it comes to Liza's wakefulness, there is no predictable rhythm to the day.

During the infusion, one nurse covers the bag containing the yellow, liquid amphotericin with black paper, explaining that it is standard practice to prevent exposure of the medicine to light, which would render it less effective. She sounds proud of her knowledge, proud of taking the extra step. But the other nurses do not cover the bag, and the inconsistency alarms us. We ask the doctors on rounds, and they say they don't know but promise to check. When the attending returns, he says that in the past, amphotericin needed to be shielded from light, but now it is manufactured differently and is more stable. The well-intentioned nurse is following out-of-date information. Can't the nurses and doctors talk to each other?!

The next time the nurse is on duty, she does not cover the bag. With her face and body language, she conveys skepticism, as if to say, *I'll follows orders, but if the medicine is ineffective, don't blame me.*

Could she be right? I imagine that all this effort, the lengthy infusions, might be useless in fighting Liza's fungal infection and that it could overwhelm her. On the other hand, I am furious at the nurse, furious at having to rely on a sprawling network of imperfectly coordinated human beings, of which she is only one small part. Then I worry that I am naïve to believe the doctor. The only way to be sure he is giving us accurate information is to go look it up myself in a medical library or on the Internet. But I don't have the time or energy. This is draining. Elena and I are working hard to keep Liza comfortable, informed, distracted, and upbeat. We are working hard to understand the medical situation, to advocate for Liza, to spare her any inconsiderate treatment, and to avoid lapses in care while simultaneously trying to keep Molly's life stable. Can't we trust the team to figure out whether the medicine is stable in light or not?

Liza needs her defenses to fight the infection. Her chemotherapy must be halted until the infection is successfully treated. Elena and I reemploy the martial metaphor to better comprehend the situation: Before, we were in a fight against sick white blood cells. But now we're being attacked from the rear by the fungi. It isn't feasible to battle on both fronts at once. The two of us so strongly identify with Liza that we speak of her illness as *our* illness, her fight as our fight—one in which we are wholly united. And yet we're painfully aware that only Liza gets the chemotherapy. I wish I could take it for her, take the entire wretched ordeal from her body into my own, and I know Elena feels the same way. When I sit by her bedside, I simultaneously feel empowered to help Liza cope with all the obstacles she faces and, at another level, utterly helpless.

※   ※   ※

On a Sunday, after almost two weeks of amphotericin completed and with two more weeks to go, I enter Liza's hospital room and find her in agony. She is lying in Elena's arms. In a whisper, Elena explains, "It began late last night. Liza was suddenly racked by horrible pain in her back and abdomen."

I watch while Liza continues to seek out a position that will bring her more comfort, pleading to be held motionless until the pain returns. She insists that we be silent or be as quiet as we can if we have to speak at all. Her whimpers are punctuated by screams. Elena and I find this more horrible than anything we've faced before. Not knowing the cause of Liza's torment fuels our anxiety. The doctors are considering a variety of possibilities: a complication from the infection, such as an abscess; an unrelated problem, such as appendicitis; a new infection. While the test results are pending, the doctors hesitate to treat Liza's pain with analgesics. Finally, the biochemistry lab reveals acute, severe pancreatitis—a known possible side effect of one of the chemotherapy medicines she's been on, L-asparaginase. If that's the cause, it will take some time to resolve because Liza has already received three intramuscular doses. By now, the compound is in her tissue and it is being released slowly, poisoning her pancreas a little at a time.

All day, Liza wants to be held. She is thirsty, but she is NPO: The gastrointestinal system should be left alone to remove any demand upon the pancreas to produce digestive enzymes. When the nurse allows ice chips, Liza asks, "If ice is frozen water, why are ice chips any better than sips of water?" No one answers this satisfactorily, and we all bristle in frustration. The doctor on call orders pain medicine (Demerol via IV) every four hours. But no extra medicine is provided if Liza's pain persists, which it does. We plead her case at the nursing station—begging for more medicine or larger doses or shorter intervals—but to no avail. On Demerol, Liza, lying on Elena, is glazed and tired, but often less than fully asleep. When awake, she is still and distant, frighteningly distant. She notices gifts dropped off by friends, but she doesn't touch them.

On Monday, the hem-onc doctors consult with the gastroenterologists, and another squad of attendings and fellows arrives to study Liza. Being in a teaching hospital has advantages in terms of brainpower, but we are drowning in doctors, many of whom begin by taking Liza's history all over again. The gastrointestinal (GI) consultants outline a professorial review of the differential diagnosis with an obsessive commitment to cover every possibility. The GI attendings seem to be preening to me, demonstrating their familiarity with the exotic and covering themselves against future second-guessing. I find it infuriating but worrying, too, lest one of the zebras they are listing will be the cause. But it seems that the entire hem-onc team believes L-asparaginase to be the culprit.

A CAT scan can assist in understanding what's going on. From the doctors' perspective, the scan is benign, quick, illuminating. But we already encountered a daylong delay some months ago waiting for one. The hospital does not have enough scanners, and there is almost always a bottleneck unless the clinical situation is critical. Unstable patients, who may have suffered a stroke or an accident and whose treatment therefore requires an immediate CAT scan, go to the head of the line. I understand the triage system; Liza's comfort isn't the top priority.

For us, it is a different matter. Liza feels sicker and is suffering more pain than any of the three of us have ever felt in our lives. She is continually nauseous. Piercing pain repeatedly breaks through the medication, and when it does, she pales, stiffens, and cries. We hunger to root out the cause and quash it.

One night as I sleep in the hospital, a nurse comes in early and tells me to have Liza ready to drink a quart of "contrast material" (barium) that tastes "like a milkshake" before going for a CAT scan. But nothing tastes good to Liza. I explain to her what she will have to do, showing her the container of liquid the nurse has brought. We wait throughout the morning, but the call does not come. Elena arrives, and we bring her up to date. Finally, upon receiving a call from the CAT scan technician, the clerk announces over the room intercom, "They will be ready for Liza soon." We tell Liza to begin drinking and encourage her to continue. She sips and sips, slowly, even though she gags on the chalky, unpleasant stuff. Now Liza is ready for the CAT scan, but it is not ready for her. The nurse and then the resident call the CAT scan staff, but they receive no clarification. The scan is delayed until the afternoon. In the afternoon, it is delayed until tomorrow.

The next morning, Liza's morning nurse, Colleen, announces that Liza is next for the scan and brings the loathsome "milkshake." An hour later, Colleen returns to say she has just learned there will be a delay; she wasn't given a reason. I dread a repetition of previous experiences when we had to wait all day for a test. Upset, having nothing to lose, and wearing my usual overnight attire—striped pants, T-shirt, and slippers—I go to the office of the chairman of the Department of Radiology and ask his secretary for an audience. She picks up the phone, then points me to his door. Despite my frazzled and disheveled appearance, or perhaps because of it, this kindly, grandfatherly gentleman interrupts his office work and asks, "How can I help you?"

"My name is Philip Lister, and my daughter Liza is an inpatient on the fifth floor. She is waiting to get a CAT scan. I know there's a bottleneck. But she's four years old, she has leukemia, and she has acute pancreatitis, probably a reaction to asparaginase, so she's NPO and in pain and in limbo being called to the scan. She's told to drink a big container of contrast, and then the scan is cancelled and she's told to drink it all over again. That went on all day yesterday, and today seems to be a repeat. I know there's a triage system with crises taking priority, but I thought you might be able to help." I am aware of the tremble in my voice as I try to be objectively succinct. He is attentive.

"I can't promise anything, but I will see what I can do." He extends his hand. "Best of luck."

A little later, they call Liza to the scan, and I feel triumphant. She is told to drink another quart of contrast material because so much time has elapsed since the original batch. Again, she sips slowly as we make our way to the scan room in the hospital basement. After another half hour waiting in the corridor, they take Liza, and the scan is done within thirty minutes.

"I'm glad they got the scan done," says Dr. Hollander, our current ward attending, stopping in with Drs. Stevens and Mueller on her late-afternoon rounds. At first I am unsure, but after a moment, I can tell she knows nothing of my visit to the radiology chair. The three of them bring Elena and me to the empty parents' lounge, a room almost always vacant except at night, when hospital aides and escorts eat and watch TV on their breaks. Reporting on the CAT scan, Dr. Hollander puts it bluntly: "Her pancreas is decimated." I can see that our doctors are shaken.

"It's—it's completely destroyed?" I choke out.

"No," Art answers—Dr. Stevens by now is Art to us. "It is not totally gone. But it is severely injured, and its resilience is being tested; how fully it will be able to function cannot yet be known. We have sharply increased Liza's pain medicine. To support her, we will give her nutrition through the IV. For now, she must stay NPO. The entire digestive tract needs to rest so that the pancreas can heal."

"So was the pancreatitis caused by the asparaginase?" I ask.

"Yes," says Dr. Hollander. "No more L-asparaginase for Liza—ever."

"Is there another medication that you add in its place?" asks Elena.

Art explains, "No. Patients are often unable to tolerate one or even two of the six chemotherapy medications. We still expect Liza to do well. We are eager for her to recover so that chemotherapy can be resumed. Although the delay to date is not worrisome, the longer the delay, the greater the risk of relapse."

With that, we break our huddle. Elena and I hold on to each other as we make our way back to Liza's room with a wobble that betrays our mix of relief (to have a diagnosis and plan), horror (at the word "decimated"), and worry. Will her pancreas recover? Will it recover soon enough to resume chemo and prevent relapse?

Just as they did on Day Zero, the doctors do not dwell on the options available in the event of relapse.

✳ ✳ ✳

Because of her pancreatitis, Liza's body becomes edematous—swollen by her weakened blood vessels weeping, oozing serum into the soft tissues of her body. Her legs and arms swell. All of her skin is puffy, and her calves bear deep impressions from the elastic tops of her slipper socks. The nurses and doctors have much more difficulty now finding veins from which to draw blood. The IV lines have to be replaced more often. When one stops working, we put Emla, a numbing cream, on several spots on her arms and hands and ask the staff to wait for the effect to take hold. Most of the veins in Liza's arms and hands are used up, leaving behind scattered bruises and distended blotches. The staff recommends a special IV—a PICC (peripherally inserted central catheter) line.

The new PICC line is large enough to support a blood transfusion, and Liza needs one. Her own blood cell production has decreased, both because of her chemotherapy and because of her acute illnesses (fungal infection followed by pancreatitis), and phlebotomy day after day also contributes to Liza's anemia. We are prepared. Organized by a family friend so close to us that we call her "Aunt Lisa," our inner circle works tirelessly to organize a network of friends and acquaintances to give blood and platelets. According to an intricate schedule, someone donates every few days, so that directed donations are always available for Liza. By organizing the donations, we reduce one small element of uncertainty, grabbing control of the situation where we can.

After a few days, Liza's pain eases its grip. Perhaps the inflamed pancreas is quieting down or the medication is controlling the pain. Only rarely is her sleep punctuated by grunts and whimpers of distress, and when that happens, extra Demerol allows her to relax into sounder sleep. Without the Broviac catheter coming out of her chest, Liza sleeps on her stomach again. In alert moments, she asks astute questions. "What did the CAT scan show?" "What did the sonogram show?" She listens carefully to our explanations. At times, she laughs, telling us that under the sway of Demerol, she has had visions of seeing "fish with hands and feet!"

* * *

Though Elena and I welcome visits from our friends, Liza views adults, especially those she does not know well, as intruders. She is surly and hardly responds to them. When she's left out of the conversation, whether Elena and I are both with her or it is only a friend and one of us, Liza becomes livid, demanding that we be quiet. "Can I please have a few minutes of silence! Please, Mommy, please!" Often Elena and I speak in murmurs or scrawl notes back and forth, as if trying to outsmart a volatile, nasty teacher. Peeved, I scribble to Elena, *I'm going to talk as loud as I want for as long as I want, and we're having as many visitors as we want. So there!* Elena chuckles, and I relax, having vented my pent-up irritation. It's another balancing act. We require some civility from Liza, but we also try to respect her wish that visits be quiet and brief. (With visits from family— Molly, the grandmothers, or the New Hampshire Listers—or from our closest friends, Liza is much less prickly.) Elena artfully creates

compromises, diffusing moments when I am too harsh or too indulg-
ing of Liza. "Lizie, Janet is here to see all of us. We'll talk with her for
a few minutes, and then we'll have a few minutes of quiet." I learn
from watching Elena, and I provide equilibrium on the rare occasion
when Elena loses hers.

One Sunday afternoon, Elena's dad, Grandpa Sumner, calls to
ask if he can visit. Because of his own poor health, he rarely goes
anywhere other than to hemodialysis three times a week. Clearly,
this visit to Liza is important to him. Using a cane to steady himself, and with Grandma Doris at his side, he shuffles into Liza's hospital room. We guide him to the easy chair next to her bed and help
him remove his overcoat. He drops into the seat. Liza, who has been
watching television, updates him. "They think I'm allergic to asparaginase—one of my chemo medicines. So I don't have to take it
anymore. It messed up my pancreas." Then, after taking some pain
medicine, she falls asleep. He switches channels to find a football
game. Chatting quietly with Elena and me while we play cards with
Molly, Doris explains, "He insisted on coming today, regardless of
the cold weather. He needed to see Liza and show his support." His
courage and poise in dealing with multiple medical problems (among
them bladder cancer, kidney failure, and severe heart disease) have
inspired us, but Sumner says that he has it much easier than Liza. "It
must be so hard to be so sick and so young." Uncharacteristically, his
eyes tear. A few moments later, he is dozing. Despite his many come-
backs, I don't believe Sumner will live much longer. The two sleep-
ers, granddaughter and grandfather, both disfigured—Liza's face
rounder, her scalp bald; Sumner's face gaunt, his hair thin—make a
sad, yet beautiful, picture.

*　*　*

After an unusually good day, Liza has another fever spike.
Twenty-four hours later, the blood culture shows a new fungal
growth. This new setback will require another course of IV amphotericin, a heftier dose this time, and of longer duration. Dr. Carter,
a resident, removes the PICC line without delay and places a new
IV in Liza's right arm. He takes us aside and acknowledges that the
IV will last only a few days. Because of the state of Liza's skin and

veins, he says, "the problem of 'access' has become huge." He consults with the head of the pediatric intensive care unit (PICU, pronounced "pick you"), who gently, carefully, inspects Liza's skin, her arms and hands, feet and legs. She strikes us as a sensitive and skilled woman. For Liza to get the multiple medicines she needs, and, if necessary, IV nutritional support, it will be helpful for there to be two points of IV access, especially because she will require the lengthy infusions of amphotericin. The doctor proposes placing a bifurcated line with two lumens in Liza's jugular vein, just under her left jaw; it would provide two IV entry ports and solve the increasingly tense problem of access. The procedure is risky, because neck veins, although large, are not as superficial as arm or leg veins, and there can be significant bleeding, but there are no safer options. If the jugular line is carefully anchored and kept clean, it can last for at least ten days.

The next day, Liza is wheeled on a gurney to the PICU, where the head of the unit performs the procedure smoothly. From the tape on Liza's skin two thin tubes emerge—one yellow, the other lime green. We are relieved that she now has a stable, reliable IV line. But we also feel assaulted. Until now, Liza's soft neck had seemed such a safe part of her body.

It disturbs her that the IV line is in a part of her body that she cannot see without a mirror. The tape used to secure the two IV tubes irritates her skin. She worries that she could damage the IV line if she moves her neck too much or scratches the itchy spots. But there is no equivalent of an arm board for her neck, no way to prevent movements of her head. We try to reassure her and to distract her, but we share her worry.

Lab tests indicate steady improvement in Liza's pancreatitis. She begins to eat some of the foods she has been craving: bagels, watermelon, small frozen waffles with syrup. One GI attending, relaxed at seeing Liza's improvement, begins to tell Elena about one of his young patients with some psychological difficulties, leading up to asking if she might be available for a referral—all in front of Liza, in fact, speaking across her bed. Elena ends the discussion by saying she isn't taking any new patients at the moment, but after he leaves, she and I look at each other with eyes wide. *Did that really just happen? Not cool at all.*

Elena structures Molly's visits with projects that both girls can work on, such as making perfume or jewelry. Nonetheless, there are lulls during which Liza becomes cranky and demands silence or Molly becomes bored and restless. Sometimes this happens as a weekend visit is coming to a close, when Molly is about to leave with one of us to begin her week at school. Elena and I explain to both of them that annoyance with each other during visits is part of being sisters, part of the strain of not being together in our own home. One such Sunday night, Liza becomes tearful after Molly leaves and tells her mother, "I have no choices anymore. I always have to do or not do what somebody else says." No wonder Liza wants to be the boss of talking. Feeling guilty, she asks if Molly will not want to come back to visit. Elena reassures her that Molly understands. That night, with Elena's encouragement, Liza apologizes to Molly on the phone for being rude and asks if she will visit again.

Molly immediately grasps what Liza needs from her. "I will be back next Saturday—definitely!"

"I'm proud of you, Mol—you're quite the impressive big sis," I tell her when we all hang up. "I hope you know that I get angry with Lizie at times, and Mommy, too." She laughs.

✳ ✳ ✳

At the hospital with Liza, I begin painting with watercolors. In the past, I occasionally drew or painted birthday cards for Elena and the girls. Now I doodle in anticipation of Valentine's Day. I paint pictures with hidden hearts in the style of Hidden Pictures in *Highlights for Children*, creating a game for the girls to find all of them. When Liza was doing poorly, watercoloring relaxed and engrossed me, especially when she slept and I could not. Immersed in the color, I'd forget that I was in the hospital for a moment. Now, with Liza feeling better, whenever I take out my paints, she is interested.

"Daddy, I love this one. How many hearts are there going to be?"

"So far, there are thirteen, but there are going to be a few more."

"Thirteen! Can I look for them yet?"

"Not yet, silly goose. Do you want to do some painting too?"

"Yes, please." Using the elevated tray that can slide across her

Serving as the tooth fairies, Elena and I happily celebrate this ordinary milestone.

* * *

"I'm feeling like I have a fever," Liza says late one afternoon at home. The thermometer registers 102 degrees. Dr. Steinherz admits Liza and starts two antibiotics. Liza's blood cultures are positive for staphylococcus, a common microbe. Again, the doctor must remove Liza's Broviac catheter, thus more needles and IVs.

This hospitalization is going to last at least two weeks, maybe more. Elena and I renew sharing a journal that we keep beside Liza's bed. We concentrate on what we can do to help her feel more comfortable and enjoy the hours of the day. We bring new movies, books, games, and foods she likes when she has any appetite. Liza's responsiveness to these efforts, her appreciation of the things we bring, lifts our spirits. And that lift we get from her fuels Elena and me to think of more we can do to give a lift to Liza. Round and round, lift begets lift, countering the sporadic sags.

There are moments when exhaustion and dread overcome me—most commonly on my nights at home after Molly is in bed. If she might be free to talk, I phone Elena. I learn that she wrestles with the same demons when she is at home. We agree that being at the hospital with Liza is easier; it involves staying busy taking care of her—everything from giving medicine to hanging out, watching a movie together. Involved with the real demands of the situation, we can keep fear at a distance. At home, fear for Liza's future, or dismay at what she is going through, seeps forward and grabs us. If I cannot reach Lainie, I call a friend. If I don't feel like talking, I snack on something crunchy or, resisting the urge to eat, I get on the exercise bike and turn on the TV. But not the news, not the dramas, not even the sports that would usually capture me. It's hard to care. I lose myself in the drone of the fan and the hum of the pedals. Or I do nothing, nothing but fret and sleep.

* * *

Molly asks to have a slumber party to celebrate turning eight. Quickly, we pull it together. I recall that the seamstress who made hats for Liza when her hair first came out also aspired to be a puppeteer. She is delighted to hear from me, and she and her partner will put on a puppet show for Molly and her friends.

The party falls on a night when Elena is scheduled to sleep over with Liza. Aunt Lisa comes over to help and stay while Elena and I change places. Our living room fills with bedrolls and sleeping bags. We rent movies and get takeout from McDonald's. The puppeteers arrive late, and although their act is not at all polished, more like a rehearsal than a show, Molly and her friends have a blast, responding to every joke as if the living room is filled with laughing gas. Afterward, I hurry to the hospital twelve blocks away so that Elena can enjoy some time with Molly and the girls; she'll make them popcorn and begin the videos. A few hours later, around ten o'clock, Lainie returns to the hospital and I go home. Lisa leaves as the girls settle in to sleep. I shepherd the girls through the night and make them a pancake breakfast.

* * *

Despite Liza's staph infection, Dr. Steinherz schedules another three-week cycle of chemotherapy. To stave off the next inevitable relapse, to maintain Liza in remission for as long as possible, chemotherapy should continue without interruption. Elena and I keep track of the prescribed agents, although we are more casual about it than we were a year ago.

One evening on my watch, our nurse, Julia, seems harried. She brings Liza's evening medicines a few hours after supper, much later than usual, near nine o'clock. Although she has not been one of our primary nurses, she knows us. Attractive, cordial, but aloof, she conducts her duties quickly, identifies the medicines she deposits on the rolling tray table, and leaves. By now, everyone knows that Liza takes her meds with Cleveth, Elena, or me.

I look over the tray and notice an unfamiliar medicine—a chemotherapy drug that Liza has never taken before. Looking in the medicine cup, something strikes me as not right. A bunch of pills are sitting there, more than I was expecting. Uncertain, I push the call button. Over the intercom, Julia, sounding rushed and irritated, asks, "Is there a problem?"

"I have a question about one of Liza's medicines."

It really is like talking to a wall when she says, "I'm quite busy, but I will come take a look when I can."

I give Liza her other medications, holding the one to the side. It is her chemotherapy, the most important one. Should I just give it to her? Other than this, we are ready to go to sleep. I decide to wait. It takes Julia an hour to arrive. We rarely have to wait for nursing help at Memorial, and never this long before. When she comes in, I explain my concern. She clarifies that she brought five pills, six milligrams each.

"Thirty milligrams doesn't sound right to me. Will you please recheck it?"

With some irritation, she agrees to do so, but she warns me again that it may take a while. Liza and I make our pre-bed bathroom trip, and then I read to her. I'm tucking her in when Julia enters the room brusquely. She takes away the medicine and returns immediately with a much smaller dose—half of one pill. Visibly tense, she says, "The correct dose is three milligrams, not thirty. Someone transcribed the order incorrectly." Abruptly, she turns and leaves.

Jesus Christ! That is horrifying! Is it okay to be mad about this? Relearning the need to be vigilant, I contain my fury, my dismay, my worry. I'm proud that I protected Liza from harm, glad that she did not receive ten times the intended dose. But what about an apology? A word of acknowledgment from Julia? Aren't we on the same team?

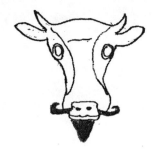

9—FINAL PREPARATIONS
November 1995

Liza shares a double room with Sasha, a twelve-year-old girl from Indiana. Elena and I feel a connection with Sasha's family. Their child and ours are both on the way to bone marrow transplant. We each have two girls; their well, younger child, Anne, is eight, Molly's age. Both of Sasha's parents work, and we seem to share similar values, if our behavior with our kids is any indication. More often than not, we keep the curtains open.

"Sasha, did you do your math homework yet," we hear, "and the reading for English?"

"Yes, Mom, I finished both, but I still have history to do tomorrow."

Liza is delighted when Sasha gives her several paintings and other creations from the playroom.

"When Anne comes to visit, let's have her meet Molly," I suggest. All the grown-ups agree. Lainie and I realize it would be a boon for all of us if Sasha and Liza are in the bone marrow transplant unit at the same time.

A few days later, Sasha needs more medical attention. The fevers for which she was admitted are recurring, despite antibiotics. Sasha feels lousy and her curtain stays drawn. Through the night, doctors come often to check on her and to draw blood. The next morning, Sasha leaves the room for a test. She does not return.

Elena sees Sasha's mother in the hall and asks, "Is Sasha okay?"

"She had to be transferred to the pediatric intensive care unit at New York Hospital." Elena hugs her.

"What happened to Sasha?" Liza asks.

"She needed to be closer to the doctors and nurses, because her infection wasn't getting better," Elena explains.

"I hope she feels better and comes back to our room," Liza says.

"Yeah. It was fun to have her here."

With Sasha's belongings gone and the bed vacant, the room seems emptier, lonelier. I feel unsettled. It was so quickly comfortable to meet this Midwestern family, such a surprise to find a warm connection, and then it was just gone—as though we'd found an oasis, but as we scooped up the first handful of water, it disappeared, desert again.

* * *

Elena and I meet with Dr. Kernan in a small classroom. At the start, we three sit in student chairs with laminate lamb-chop-shaped tablet arms for note-taking.

"Of the relatives on Phil's father's side who agreed to be tested, none are matches," begins Nancy. "I see no benefit in pursuing any further testing of living relatives. A donor from the national registry has been identified, and procedures with that donor are going well. I am given only limited information about the donor, but I am told the donor is reliable and enthusiastic."

"Enthusiastic?" I repeat without thinking.

"Yes, enthusiastic," she confirms. "The donor matches Liza in five out of the six chromosome sites we test. While we still hope for a six-out-of-six match, this match is very good. If all goes well, we will proceed with the transplant."

She goes to the blackboard and outlines our lesson in bone marrow transplantation. "The first step is radiation—TBI, stands for total body irradiation. That's followed by chemotherapy. Together they will destroy all of Liza's bone marrow—healthy and cancerous cells alike. It will cause you anxiety to see Liza's blood counts plummet to zero, it always does, but that's what we want to happen. And we'll be covering her with lots of medications to prevent infections—bacterial, fungal, or viral. At that point, Liza will receive the donor marrow. We look for the donor cells to 'engraft' over the next few days. If they do, it means that they take up residence in Liza's bone marrow space. And then they will start to produce new, healthy blood cells, and her blood counts will rise gradually toward normal levels."

After we get the overview, Nancy explains that the donor's marrow can be treated one of several ways and that the way it is prepared is determined by computer as part of the research protocol. She then continues, "Chemotherapy and radiation will involve a variety of side effects and long-term risks. The radiation may cause a deficiency in growth hormone, hypothyroidism, neurological damage, cataracts, and cancers—called 'secondary cancers'—in adulthood. Infertility is highly likely." Elena and I both shudder. "Like all transplant patients, Liza will have to be monitored closely for years by a team that will include a neuropsychologist to assess any impairment in cognition or learning disabilities as well as an endocrinologist."

"Did you say infertility?" I ask.

"While it's not absolutely certain, almost always the ovarian function is knocked out by radiation. I know it's upsetting. Of course, we wouldn't be doing any of this by choice." We nod.

She goes on, "I've been thinking about separation. The usual policy of the transplant unit is that patients stay in their cubicle alone— with visits, of course, but not constant companionship. But in getting to know Liza and your family, I've concluded that Liza will do better if she is not separated from you two. I have appealed to the committee in charge of procedures and won their approval so that one of you can stay with Liza as you have been doing on the regular ward."

"That's a huge relief. We really appreciate you advocating for us, Nancy," says Elena.

"Is there any way we can thank our enthusiastic donor?" I ask.

"You aren't allowed to exchange names, but with that restriction, you can write a note, which will be screened to be sure there is no identifying information and delivered to her."

"Her!" I notice.

"Him or her." She smiles. "But this policy is to protect people on both sides from an emotional entanglement that may turn out to be unwanted. After one year, the donor has the choice to have his or her name revealed."

I look at Elena and shrug. "We can understand that."

* * *

Elena learns from one of the nurses that Sasha has died from an infection. The supports and medicines that the intensive care unit offered could not save her. So we won't be meeting her sister, won't be getting the two families together after all. I search for a reason to think that what happened to Sasha cannot happen to Liza, some reason to think that Liza is less vulnerable or that Elena and I are better protectors. I can find no such reason. Our best efforts to take care of Liza can protect her only so much. We cannot eliminate her vulnerability any more than Sasha's parents could.

If Liza asks about Sasha, what will we say? We value being honest with Liza, but it would frighten her to hear the truth. It has frightened us. My intuition is that Liza will not ask, but our tentative plan if she does is to stall, to say that we aren't sure what has happened to Sasha though we can try to find out, buying some time so Elena and I can figure out what we want to say, taking into account how Liza seems at that time.

* * *

Dr. Steinherz feels it is safe to insert a new Broviac, this one with three lumens. The familiar foot-long catheter coils away from Liza's chest before it trifurcates, the branches ending in colored ports— red, white, and blue.

"How long will *this* Broviac last?" she asks, voicing an unspoken question that Elena and I have as well.

Elena acknowledges, "It's hard to count on these darn Broviacs, isn't it?"

"We're on our third one already!" Liza says.

"Well, Lizie," I note, "you know the doctors wanted you to have a three-lumen Broviac for the transplant anyway. And this one looks like it is by far the best. We hope it will last until you are all done with treatment and don't need a Broviac anymore."

Each Broviac has become a charmed object—at once an extension of Liza's body that has been altered by illness, a source of vulnerability to infection, and the wizardry of modern medicine that spares Liza many needles and IVs. We love it, we hate it, we depend upon it, we dread its malfunction.

Now that Liza feels better and is able to move her arms around without constant caution for IVs, she wearies of being in the hospital, of tubes and wounds and manipulations. "I'm tired of being in Memorial Sloan Kettering. I'm here so much, it feels like I live here. They should call this place the 'house-pital.'"

On Sunday, we bring in the Sunday *New York Times*. Liza vents her anger by tearing up sections from the paper. I am about to object, but I catch a look from Elena, a look that says this is harmless and we should support Liza venting. At first Liza uses scissors and then puts them aside to use both hands to rip and crumple page after page. Amid the shredded mess, she declares, "I wish they would get on with getting me well. It's been a whole year!"

When her storm subsides, she becomes giddy, then shifts to playing imaginatively, inaudibly, with her little plastic toy figures. She emerges from her play with a thought: "Let's make Molly a tie-dyed sweatshirt. I know she wants one."

*   *   *

On a Thursday evening, Liza and I are in the hospital playroom, and she's playing with a teddy bear with a Broviac. Sharone appears. Our dear friend and colleague was Elena's classmate in training. As both are youthful, petite brunettes, they have been mistaken for each other frequently over the years by those who don't know them well. We have the big playroom almost to ourselves. Sharone makes conversation easily with Liza, telling her about a recent discussion she and her husband, Jeff, had with their two boys, one a little older and the other a little younger than Liza.

"The boys really want a pet, and Jeff and I are willing—if the boys will take care of it. The problem is in choosing the pet. Of all things, the boys really want an iguana. But I did some research and found out that iguanas can grow to six feet!"

Liza chuckles.

"We told them they absolutely cannot keep an iguana once it is longer than three feet. But of course the boys don't want to get a pet that they'll have to give away. We talked about a dog, but Jeff and I don't think they're old enough to take care of a dog. As for cats, Jeff is allergic."

Liza points to me. "Daddy is too."

"Hamsters and guinea pigs are in the running, but they can be noisy at night, they have to stay in their cages most of the time, and their cages can get smelly." Sharone's voice and face show her perplexity.

After a moment, Liza says, "Do you want to know what I would do?" She waits for Sharone to reply.

"Yes, Liza, I certainly do."

Steadfastly looking at Sharone, Liza explains, "I would get the iguana. And I would enjoy it in the time I had it. The way I would do that is by knowing that one day I wouldn't have it." Sharone and I exchange glances to confirm that we both really heard what we think we heard from this five-year-old. Liza notices the pause and adds, "The iguana is the one they really want."

❖ ❖ ❖

On the Monday of Thanksgiving week, Dr. Steinherz comes to Liza's room. "Liza, let's get you home," he announces.

She beams and asks, "When?"

"I think you should pack up now." He smiles and gives us some final instructions before leaving.

"I hope they don't change their minds," Liza says.

We schedule a visit to the nineteenth floor right after the holiday to meet with Megan, the head nurse of the bone marrow transplant unit.

❖ ❖ ❖

The nineteenth floor is a zone of hope and danger. Bringing Molly and Liza, we make a family expedition. We take the express elevator and wait for the head nurse to meet us. Megan appears, a tall woman with short blond hair. Like a towering Iowa cornstalk, she evokes bright sun and blue skies. She radiates strength. Alert and attentive to the girls' needs, she immediately notices their uncertainty as they step into this new place that might as well be Mars. Taking them under her wing, she shows them the mobile racks laden with supplies (booties, gowns, caps). She outlines the procedures to minimize the presence of germs—lengthy handwashing, sterile garb—but because these steps are not required for today's visit, Megan does not belabor the details. She takes care to avoid overloading the kids with information they need not retain.

After some ordinary handwashing, Megan leads us into a room designated "dirty"—meaning that a patient recently vacated the room and it has been cleaned only superficially and not fully sterilized. To me, the bright little cubicle seems cleaner than clean. From the entrance, covered by a curtain—not a door—we face a large, glorious window that is the width of the far wall and that offers our eyes the feast of a big, clear sky. Looking down, I see the slow-moving East River, which changes directions with the tides, and its occasional boat traffic. The left wall is white, with small holes like a pegboard. This wall hides a huge HEPA (high-efficiency particulate air) filter; filtered air enters the room through the holes. The other two walls are Plexiglas, solid except for one hole, six inches in diameter, near the head of the bed. From its stand outside the room, the intravenous machinery will send three different fluids through spiraled tubes to the three ports of Liza's Broviac. Also outside this wall, bins will hold our sterilized belongings. The nurses, doctors, janitors, and other staff—all the traffic of the unit is visible, though curtains can be pulled to reduce the noise and distraction of the people passing by.

After bringing us here, showing us about, and answering our questions, Megan leaves us to acclimate ourselves and make sense of the place. The important feature for the girls is the television suspended from the ceiling and its remote control. There is minimal furniture—one chair and ottoman, a sliding tray on wheels, wheeled wire racks for holding sterile medical supplies. Liza and Molly get on the hospital bed, which lies alongside the air filtration wall and faces the window. They check out the TV and celebrate when they find Nickelodeon and the Disney Channel. They discover the buttons that regulate the bed's various positions. With merriment, and more harmoniously than usual, Molly and Liza take turns raising and lowering the head of the bed, the foot of the bed, and then the entire bed.

They make us edgy by raising the bed "so high!"—even with the side rails raised. Giggling, they get onto their knees and pretend to tee-ter atop the bed. Elena and I act out our roles as anxious parents, dis-traught and alarmed at seeing that "the girls are so high!" We ham it up: "Girls, come down from there, please—it's too high!" or "Girls, get that bed back down here this instant!" or "Hang on, girls; we've called the fire department and they'll be right over to get you down." Peals of laughter rain down from our rebels.

Twenty minutes later, Megan peeks in—our cue to gather our-selves. We issue the girls a two-minute warning. Liza whines, "I want to stay a little while longer." The giggles ebb. The spell is broken.

Before we leave, Megan shows us to a conference room, where we sit for a few minutes. Do we have any questions?

Liza asks, "Will I be able to lick Mommy?"

"No, I'm afraid not, not until you leave."

Liza looks deflated for a moment and then turns to Elena, who is seated beside her. She says, "I'll just have to get my licks in now." Like a little puppy, she gives Elena some licks on the cheek and nose and then turns to me and gives me a few. Molly laughs and covers up as Liza turns to her.

Megan shows us some brochures and coloring books and other printed material to help children understand BMT. We pack them up, glad to have the material. Going down in the elevator, I realize that the question that occurred to me (and no doubt to Elena) from the start of our visit may also have occurred to Molly and Liza: How did that room we just left come to be empty—which of the two pos-sible ways?

*   *   *

That same week after Thanksgiving, on the morning of the mar-row harvest, we meet Dr. Fry, an attending on the transplant team doing harvests this month. When we meet, Liza, in a hospital gown, is lying on a gurney ready for the operating room. Dr. Fry, in surgical garb, including hat, tries to establish rapport by picking up the bean-bag cow Liza has brought with her and talking of her own daughter's beanbag collection. But Liza bristles. Sullen, she avoids eye con-tact and does not respond to the doctor's comments and questions.

She turns to Elena and protests, "She's got my cowie!" Out of tune with Liza's temperament, or annoyed by her unresponsiveness, Dr. Fry keeps trying to jolly her into good humor, all the while handling her beanbag. Only when Liza begins to protest loudly and is on the verge of tears does she put down the cow. She apologizes to Liza in a perfunctory and scornful manner, then turns matters over to the anesthesiologist, who begins to administer the IV medication that renders Liza woozy. The aides wheel the gurney into the OR, and then Elena and I have to leave. Though the contact with Dr. Fry lasted only a few minutes, it leaves us all feeling sour, including Dr. Fry herself.

After the procedure, Elena and I go to Liza in the recovery room. She wakes in a wild confusion; her irrationality and anger last for a difficult hour. After she returns to her usual self, with large bandages on her sore haunches, we head home by midday.

*   *   *

Two days later, I bring Liza back to the hospital for her consultation with the Radiation Department. The secretary ushers us into a small examination room. After a few minutes, a young resident wearing a white jacket over green scrubs enters and introduces himself. Scarcely acknowledging Liza's presence, he interviews me on her medical history. Like a turtle, Liza, totally quiet, seems to shrink into her shell as she hears me review the broad strokes of her illness.

"Have you looked at her chart?" I ask. I can hear the exasperation in my voice, and I am pretty sure that he does too. I hate that Liza has withdrawn.

"No, I didn't," he says.

He leaves. Soon another young doctor, a more senior resident in a longer white coat, knocks and enters. He repeats the exact same interview, questioning me and ignoring Liza, who looks tinier. These doctors seem to give no consideration to what Liza must feel sitting beside me while I speak to strangers about her complex, tortuous medical history. All this could be done without her being here, but I can think of no way to recommend that now. As much as I don't want to do these interviews in front of Liza, I definitely don't want to leave her alone in the cramped exam room by going elsewhere to review her history with the doctors.

Following his redundant interview, the resident shifts gears. In what he evidently believes is an important and helpful manner, he offers information about the short- and long-term side effects of radiation. He launches into a dutiful, semi-automatic listing of potential medical problems, the ones Dr. Kernan told us about, including secondary tumors and infertility. He is totally insensitive to Liza, to whether it is appropriate for a five-year-old to hear this. As soon as I see the trajectory of his comments, I interrupt.

"You need to stop. I want to speak to your attending." Flustered, he realizes that I am serious, and he goes to find one.

"Daddy, what is going on?" Liza looks up at me, her hazel eyes wide open, baffled.

"I thought those two doctors were not very thoughtful, so I'd like to speak with someone in charge. I don't think you need to hear about *every* possible thing that can go wrong, do you?"

"No!" she declares, and laughs quietly.

When the attending, Dr. Randolph, enters the room, I ask Liza to wait a moment and I step out into the hall with him.

"Do you think that my five-year-old daughter needs to hear right now—a few days before she receives a bone marrow transplant—about the likelihood that she will be sterile or have a future cancer or any other problem because of this treatment that she will have to undergo imminently?" I started speaking calmly, but by the time I get to the end of the sentence, I can hear a fiery tremble in my voice. I take a breath. "How about if you speak with me quickly in private, while Liza waits, or I can come back without her."

I see his face shift as understanding dawns on him.

"I am truly sorry about that." As if trying to be economical with time in consideration for me, he hurries and begins to cite statistics for the risk of lymphoma and other tumors in the decades ahead.

"Again, I have to interrupt you." I pause to gather my wits and to look for a way to penetrate. "We are not here out of choice."

Abashed, he assents and gives me his card. "Go back in with your daughter. I'll get some material you can take with you."

He returns in a couple of minutes. He knocks.

"Hello, Liza." She looks up and allows him to take her hand to shake. "I'm sorry that you had to come over to the hospital an extra time today. Your dad spoke to me, and we're going to try to keep it as short a visit as we can." Handing me some booklets, he says, "Here is the information you and your wife can look over. If there are any questions, just give me a call."

With that, Dr. Randolph leads us down a corridor and around a corner, through an enormous vault-like door to the radiation machinery. He introduces us to the technicians who will perform Liza's "radiation simulation," and he leaves.

Liza is put in a harness-like framing contraption made of clear plastic panels. Measurements are taken along various portions of Liza's torso and head. The technicians explain that they want to be able to put Liza into this structure in exactly the same position from one session to the next. While they conduct this laborious process, I sit beside Liza and read to her. Cooperatively, she stands now one way, now another. Two technicians confer to be sure Liza's position is correct. When they agree, they note the measurements. One technician uses a permanent ink pen to mark Liza with two dots on the front of her chest and one dot on her back just below the neck in the midline. These dots will serve as reference marks, allowing the staff to place Liza properly when she returns for treatment in a week and a half.

"Why do the marks need to be permanent?" Liza asks me in a voice both doleful and curious.

I ask the technician with the pen. He replies that the marks need to last reliably.

Liza asks him, "Will they ever go away?"

He says the marks will diminish over time, although they may never totally vanish. I add that they will get very tiny and maybe they will disappear—after all, she is going to grow up to have a much taller, bigger body.

In this modern world, can't scientists come up with ink that fades away after a month or two? I wonder that no one seems to care. Is it that tough guys shouldn't care about a few dots? But this is my child's skin, and I do care. Her skin already bears many marks of her experience that could not be avoided. I am so angry, angry about the

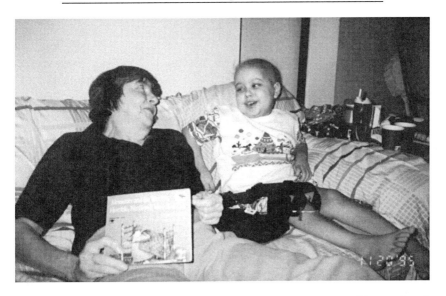

With Nanny, Liza considers *Alexander and the Terrible, Horrible, No Good, Very Bad Day*, November 20, 1995.

insensitivity we have encountered today, angry that I cannot better protect her. But as the technicians continue to mark and measure, my anger does no good.

✵ ✵ ✵

Elena takes Molly shopping for a desk worthy of her station as a student in the second grade. During a stop for soda, Molly spies a small stuffed cow, different from any of the ruminants Liza already possesses. She buys it with her own money for Liza to take with her to the transplant unit. Receiving the cow, Liza hugs it tenderly, then dances around with it and sings a variation on the familiar dreidel song, which Molly taught her:

> *Cowie, Cowie, Cowie,*
> *I made you out of love*
> *And when you're playful and ready,*
> *Oh, Cowie, I will play.*
> *Cowie, Cowie, Cowie,*
> *I made you out of love*
> *And when you're playful and ready,*
> *Oh, Cowie, I will love.*

Molly excitedly carries out our suggestion that she make a tape recording of a few of Liza's favorite stories so that Liza can listen to Molly reading to her while she is in the unpleasant vault-like radiation room. No one will be allowed in with Liza. Molly's voice is our best idea for providing Liza some companionship.

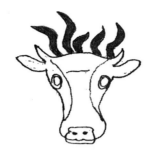

10—Transplant

December 1995–February 1996

We must change our ways. No more filling Liza's hospital room with familiar things from home. Stringent guidelines limit what is allowed on the bone marrow transplant unit. Nothing goes into Liza's room unless it has been sterilized. Most items must leave the room within forty-eight hours to be recleaned. In advance, we submit clothes, books, and other things for Liza to the head nurse, who sends them for sterilization; the items return in vacuum-sealed plastic envelopes. Shrewdly, Elena anticipates what Liza may want, allowing us to have rotations of pajamas, slipper socks, underwear, stuffed animals, games, and toys on hand.

The initially bizarre and elaborate procedure to enter Liza's cubicle quickly becomes ordinary. In the hallway outside of the unit, I cover my shoes with blue booties, my head with an elasticized mesh blue cap, my nose and mouth with a light blue mask that unfolds to fit snugly under my chin and tie in back. On entering the unit, I select a periwinkle robe and gloves from the equipment rack, each in sterile wrapping. As if prepping now for surgery, I step to a sink and begin "scrubbing in" by popping open a prewrapped soapy sponge complete with nail file. Awkwardly at first, I control the sink's water flow with foot pedals. I scrub methodically from fingertips to forearms to above the elbows—each body segment receiving twenty strokes with the sudsy sponge—before rinsing carefully so that suds go down the arms from the fingers to the elbows, never up. When done, I hail a gowning partner—a nurse or aide in the vicinity—who assists me, and with a tricky maneuver, I get my hands into my sterile gloves. Lastly, my helper holds aside the curtain that covers the entrance, and without touching it, I enter the room.

Each time I come into the room in these first days, I am struck by the oddity of our situation. Wearing her pajamas, Liza sits on her bed or in her chair. She can see only my eyes because the rest of my body is covered by all the protective gear. But after talking with Liza and hugging her, or when she sits on my lap, this alien feeling fades and often vanishes. When Elena and I visit together, it is alluring to see my wife completely covered except for her eyes. Sensing that I am intrigued by her hiddenness, she winks at me!

We learn that the room is cleanest at the wall-sized filter and that it is "dirty" at the curtained entryway. The entire room is on a clean-to-dirty gradient from one side to the other. Because the floor is not sterile, anything that falls on it must be removed per the unit's ditty: *"Touch the floor—out the door!"* In these first few days, we learn from our errors. A mindless touch to one's face means leaving the room to scrub all over again—unless one chooses to wear double gloves (very sweaty) and can then discard the sullied pair and still be safe. So, in short order, we revise our habits and control our hands.

Liza leaves the unit only to undergo total body irradiation. It is as we were told last week it would be, as we discussed with Liza. "Let's think through what is in store for us tomorrow. Sometime in the morning, we will take you to the radiation treatment. They will line you up in the frame like they did the other day. We will stay with you until they start the treatment. Then we will have to leave, but we will be able to talk to you and hear you. We will put on the tape of Molly reading stories to you." Elena and I fill in the gaps for each other.

Liza fills in gaps for both of us, asking, "I wonder if the same technicians we met last week will be there?"

Thinking ahead helps us feel calmer. When the treatment begins, the intercom is turned on.

"We're right here," we chime in. We hate to think she might feel alone or scared. Liza listens to Molly on tape. The radiation machinery whirs loudly.

At an intermission, we reenter the room, and the technicians work together to rotate Liza, confirming the location of her dots and the configuration of the plastic frame. Elena and I chat with Liza while she is realigned. I rewind Molly's tape to go back a few lines in the story under way. This time Liza faces a blank wall. She comments, "They should have some sort of picture on the wall, so patients could look at something interesting," adding, "And the painter could be you, Daddy—one of your landscapes!"

After the fourth and final round, Liza returns to her cubicle on nineteen, where she will remain until after the transplant. She receives maximum doses of chemotherapy over the next two days. To reduce ordinary bacteria in her gastrointestinal system, she takes "gut meds," medicine to kill the "gut flora." The liquid medication, taken several times each day, tastes foul—so bad that the nurses make a point of warning us it is horrible, and Liza confirms it. Specially prepared meals appear on sterilized cardboard trays, but Liza has little appetite now.

For bed baths, we use soap with a strong antibacterial formulation. Liza wants Cleveth to give them, or Mommy when Cleveth is absent. Even though the robed and masked bath-giver holds the washcloth in latex-covered hands, Cleveth and Elena enjoy a tender intimacy with Liza. She usually relaxes completely, often becoming chatty or silly. After her bath, she sometimes becomes "Baby Lizie" for a spell—something we are accustomed to at home on occasion—communicating wordlessly, only with little grunts and coos, with an imploring look on her face, her lips pursed in a duck-like expression, a glint in her eye, until she gets the snuggles and hugs she wants.

Here on nineteen, the first times Liza uses the commode in her cubicle, she is tense and self-conscious, looking around when she hears noises from the unit to see who might be able to see her. There is no bathroom for her. She asks Elena or me to sit beside her, to shield her from anyone at the entryway seeing her. But she quickly accommodates to the situation and becomes engrossed in television, ignoring intrusive sounds. Beneath the commode seat is a small basin lined with a plastic bag. As soon as Liza is done, the adult with her picks up the plastic bag, careful not to spill any of its contents, ties a knot at the top, and signals for a nurse to remove it from the room. Liza's excretions have to be analyzed regularly. Nurses mix three ointments to make "butt paste"; after Liza has a bowel movement, we must apply some to her backside.

Inside the entrance to Liza's room, one narrow shelf swivels from the wall—the dirty shelf, where nonsterilized items can stay. Twice a day, the shelf is cleaned with alcohol. Liza's tape player sits there, loaded with her favorite lullaby cassette, *'Til Their Eyes Shine*, an anthology of songs by a dozen female singers, including some of Lainie's and my favorites, among them Laura Nyro, the McGarrigle sisters, Carole King singing "If I Didn't Have You to Wake Up To," and Mary Chapin Carpenter singing "Dreamland."

"They're all my favorites," Liza says as she listens to the tape when she goes to sleep. Because hospital customs often interfere with sound sleep, she may restart the tape when she stirs, sometimes playing it often during the course of a single night.

Weakened, tired, and achy, Liza spends less time sitting alone and more time melted on a parent's lap. When it's my turn to stay overnight, she sometimes asks to be on my lap for the entire night. Sitting on the lounge chair, I extend my feet to the footstool; Liza stretches out with her back to my chest. She seems to hunger for the contact, as do I. I treasure the sight and sound and smell and feel of her, close, despite my robe and mask and gloves. The weight of her.

Chemotherapy makes her nauseous despite strong antinausea medication. Gut meds and the radiation cause bouts of diarrhea that arrive with little warning. When they began, Liza would leave the commode only to hurry back minutes later. Now she sits on the commode for long spells. Many minutes pass between peeing and pooping, but she has a feeling of urgency and prefers to get comfortable and keep sitting there.

Books and television, her main enjoyments now, entertain her whether she is on her bed, sitting in a chair, or on the commode. We don't get the Disney Channel at home, so here it provides a special alternative to her other favorites on Nickelodeon or PBS: *Rugrats*, *Rupert*, and *Wishbone*; and Nick at Nite's selection of old TV shows such as *I Love Lucy* and *Bewitched*. Liza's capacity to immerse herself in story, evident since she was two, seems particularly fortunate now. Engrossed this way, she resembles any other kid enjoying a favorite show; she even resembles herself before leukemia. I wonder if she ever forgets where she is and why. Even if she doesn't, her captivation by *Mister Rogers' Neighborhood* or *Snow White and the Seven Dwarfs* seems to soften the myriad requirements and intrusions of illness.

When not watching television, Liza turns her concentration and imagination to books. We cannot clutter her room with a stack of picture books, so we get longer books and send them to be sterilized. If we handle them carefully, we are allowed to keep them in her room for a week, and we aim to finish them within that time. Elena and I read separate books to Liza, so she has two going at any given time. Elena reads *The Chronicles of Narnia* by C.S. Lewis and *Half Magic* and related tales by Edward Eager. I pick favorites I read to Molly: *The BFG* and *Charlie and the Chocolate Factory* by Roald Dahl; three by E.B. White (*Charlotte's Web, Stuart Little, The Trumpet of the Swan*); and the books of L. Frank Baum, beginning with a large deluxe edition of *The Wizard of Oz*. The momentum of each story captivates Liza. She entrances us with her requests, uttered variously, depending on the moment. Sometimes she coaxes us softly to "read—read—read," a few more pages; sometimes she hollers, "READ—READ—READ!" I feel as if I'm her coachman, urging at her behest our team of horses to go from walk to trot to canter to gallop, always to go a little farther and a little faster. Invariably, we finish the books in time.

Liza interrupts the stories at will. When she notices a word outside her ken, she asks for a definition, an explanation. Sharing the meaning of words is delicious for Elena and me. Liza turns new words around and compares them to words she knows, until she has a firm grasp and ownership of the new. She also interrupts to muse on the direction the story is taking—how it differs from what she expected, how a character here reminds her of a character from another story, how she hopes a remedy will appear for a character lost or in a jam.

When the peach flattens Aunt Sponge and Aunt Striker with a crunch in *James and the Giant Peach*, Liza raises her hands in triumph. "Hurray! Hurray! Can you read that part again, Daddy?"

On the way to Oz, when the Lion falls asleep in the field of poppies, Liza says, "There's got to be a way to wake him up again, some medicine to break the effect of the poppies." Later, when Dorothy vanquishes the Wicked Witch and frees the Winkies, Liza anticipates, "I bet the Winkies will be able to rescue the Tin Man and the Scarecrow!" She nods with pleasure when they do.

If we flag, Liza asks, "Please, a few more minutes." Then, to help herself tolerate a break from the story, she steels herself, insisting that the final two pages—and it must be a full two pages from top left to bottom right—be read without any interruption. "No interrupting, no nothing, please, okay, not even to explain anything about what it is, what it isn't, who it is, who it isn't, the thing it is, the thing it isn't, the kind of thing it is, the kind of thing it isn't, no interrupting, no nothing, okay?!" Sometimes this becomes an incantation, part of the ritual for putting the book away, spoken so quickly that her words blur into indecipherability, leaving only a short musical breeze. All the same, I know to respond with a firm "Okay!"

✳   ✳   ✳

Every morning, blood is taken through Liza's Broviac, and every afternoon, the cell counts are posted by the door. Over the course of several days, her white cell count plummets to zero. The expected death of Liza's marrow is terrifying yet exciting. Liza receives red cell and platelet transfusions every few days. Our friends continue a stream of directed donations to the hospital blood bank.

The donor's bone marrow becomes ready on a Wednesday evening when I am staying with Liza. On December 20, six days after arriving on the nineteenth floor, we are told to expect that Dr. Molloy, a fellow we have never met before, will arrive after dinner. Liza sits on my lap, her back to my chest, listening to me read *Black Beauty* by Anna Sewell, when Dr. Molloy appears at 10:00 p.m. Our excruciating waiting is at an end. He suits up and comes into the room with Debbie, an experienced and exceptionally kind nurse from the unit who is working with us tonight. He seems on edge, influenced by the import of the event at hand. Briefly, Dr. Molloy tries to make small talk with Liza and me, but she wants none of it. In answer to my question, the doctor acknowledges that we will not see him again. He focuses on his technical task.

In his careful technique, am I seeing a slight tremulousness, or is that my own insides trembling? I cannot tell, but I am glad to sense that he appears to know what he's doing. He fills a syringe larger than any we have seen before—like a turkey baster, but wider—with clearish liquid. This is the donor's marrow. With Debbie's assistance, he connects it to one of the three IV lines that connect to Liza's Broviac. Infusing the marrow material into her blood allows the donated cells to reach Liza's now-unpopulated marrow space and to set up residence there. He glances at the clock and times the infusion, careful to go slowly, pushing only a few cc's each minute, to be sure Liza does not have an allergic reaction.

As the infusion—the long-sought, precious bone marrow transplant—begins, Debbie, with all good intention, says to Liza, "Isn't this wonderful?!"

Liza murmurs a muffled assent, but she avoids Debbie's eyes.

She tries again, "Isn't this great to get the new marrow?"

But Liza becomes more sunken and muted, turtle-like. Debbie bends down to ask, "Liza, is anything the matter?"

"No," Liza says, frowning.

Debbie, who usually enjoys an easygoing, humor-filled rapport with Liza, seems baffled and a little hurt. Feeling Liza's shoulders tense and hunched, seeing her eyebrows drawn down and in toward each other, I sense that she is overcome by the event at hand. I try to put this into words for both Debbie and Liza.

"I think it's a lot to handle just now, and it seems like it has been a long wait."

Despite the vagueness of this statement, Debbie registers understanding. She touches Liza's shoulder gently, saying, "Okay, sweetie."

I share the excitement that Debbie voiced, but I also feel for Liza. The wonder and enormity of this event—of making it this far, finding a matched donor, and having the transplant—has an unspeakable underside: If this doesn't work, Liza will die. While the infusion continues, I read *Black Beauty* aloud. After fifteen minutes, the infusion is completed. Dr. Molloy packs up his equipment and puts all of the wrappings, vials, and syringe into the appropriate receptacles. He wishes us well. When he and Debbie leave, Liza relaxes.

"That was hard for you, wasn't it?" I ask.

"Very," she acknowledges tersely.

"Was the waiting hard?"

"Very!"

"Were you worried that the doctor was going to do something more to you?"

"Well, I knew he wasn't going to do a bone marrow test, but I thought he might do something else that would hurt."

"And what about Debbie?" I ask.

"Debbie was too..." Liza begins to gesticulate, searching for the right word: "...happy."

I could not say it any better. It is too soon to celebrate—as if celebrating prematurely could usher in disappointment or jinx the project.

"Am I supposed to feel different now?" she asks.

"No, the transplant shouldn't make you feel different right away. As the new marrow makes new blood cells, you will be feeling stronger, but we weren't expecting you to feel anything right away. They were just being very careful to be sure you didn't have a bad reaction, like when you get a blood transfusion. Were you worried it would?"

"Uh-huh!"

"Does it seem weird to get the important transplant we've been waiting for and not to feel any different?"

"Uh-huh!"

The next day, Dr. Kernan drops by to acknowledge the momentous event and to monitor the daily cell counts. The donor has sent us a card, which Nancy gives to us. The front of the beautiful, rectangular card shows a picture of the beasts of creation. In the center is a stately elephant with proud wide ears, flanked by lion and peacock on the left, giraffe, hippo, and seal on the right. Bear, fox, ape, and zebra join the group portrait under a wide, vast, deep blue sky. A few scattered stars gleam. Behind the elephant's left ear is a small crescent moon. All the animals look unwaveringly at the reader.

To the Recipient and Family,

Hello. I would just like you to know that I am packing as much love as I can into my marrow so hopefully, I pray it helps. As I held my three-year-old son last night my heart went out to you. I really feel with a lot of love and faith—this makes a difference—

—Life will be better.

Please, if you could, in the future when times have settled down a bit, get in touch through whatever means to let me know your summer plans and enjoyments to come. Wishing you life and love in 1996.

May God be with you.

Sincerely,

The name has been snipped out. Reading it, I weep, as does Elena when I pass it to her. I offer to read it to Lizie, and she listens, rapt. When she gave us the card, Nancy confirmed that the donor is a woman, as the text and handwriting suggest. I am taken with the donor's idea of love packed into the marrow to make it more effective. Nancy reminds us that we may not learn one another's names for one year. After that, if both parties agree, the names can be revealed. Careful not to use names, I write a letter back to this stranger, expressing our love and gratitude, and our optimism.

We notice that the donor mentions her faith. Neither Elena nor I subscribe to any organized religion, though we take some vicarious pleasure in the donor's belief. Mia, the Taiwanese laundress on our block, tells us she prays for Liza and urges us to do likewise. With her raised eyebrow, she cautions us to take her advice seriously, rather than be sorry later. Both my father and father-in-law grew up in Orthodox Jewish homes, and finding them constricting and oppressive, both rebelled and declared themselves atheists, men of science, not illusion. Elena and I each felt attracted to the worldview of secular humanism espoused by our fathers. Nonetheless, when my yoga instructor guides a meditation at the start and end of class, I find wisdom and solace in the notion that the physical world is all an illusion—that there must be another plane, a spiritual plane, more enduring than anything physical, at the core of existence.

❊ ❊ ❊

Within a week of the transplant, white cells appear in Liza's blood. Almost every day, the white cell count creeps upward. By the second week, there is evidence of platelet production. This news means that the donor's marrow cells have engrafted and are producing new cells. The graft can still fail, but the early results are exhilarating. In the third week of Liza's stay, having waited our turn, we receive a "picture-phone." The old-fashioned device consists of two parts. One stays in Liza's room, the other goes home. Now our nightly good-night calls include sending pictures as well as talking. We do not, as we had imagined, see the people at the other end in motion. Rather, someone on one end poses, presses a button, and the camera sends a still image to the video monitor at the other end of the line; then the reverse—the recipient sends a picture back. Molly and Liza have great fun with this, and Elena and I get involved too. Making funny faces brings out the buffoon in each of us. But sometimes Liza feels weak and achy by the end of the day and doesn't respond to Molly's comical poses, and then Mol ends up disappointed and concerned.

* * *

Cleveth has been highly reliable, but now I see signs of strain. Liza sometimes lets loose on her. "Stop it, Cleveth. I don't want to have the lozenge now. Let me be! Leave me alone!" Our little girl's fury can wound deeply. We encourage Cleveth to be firm and tell us when Liza behaves poorly, but she almost never complains, and never about Liza. When Elena or I ask how she is doing, she says, "I'm okay." She doesn't open up to us, but still, she appears more burdened. She tells Elena she is looking into nursing and hopes to go back to school part-time. This is a natural choice, as babysitting Liza has drawn close to nursing. Elena writes a recommendation to accompany Cleveth's application to a nursing program. We aren't sure whether Cleveth really will pursue it or when the program might begin. We admire her interest, but we hope she won't abandon us.

* * *

Is that a rash on Liza's leg? There is definitely a red area, and she says it is a little itchy. We point it out to the doctors each morning, but they do not seem worried. One fellow says, "It might be a reaction to one of the medicines. We'll watch it."

I ask, "Could it be an early sign of graft-versus-host disease?"

"There is a chance," Nancy says, "but at present, the rash is minor."

We inquire, what other signs of GVHD might we be looking for? Other than rash, the doctors cite diarrhea. But nothing is simple in that regard; at this stage, most patients have diarrhea caused from the gut meds or the lingering effects of radiation.

But the rash on Liza's leg does not go away. New rashes appear and itch fiercely, particularly on her hands and feet. The staff tells us with confidence now that this is indeed the rash of acute graft-versus-host disease. The first treatments to try are steroids, with which Liza has had extensive experience, and cyclosporine, a potent immune suppressant, with many possible side effects—hypertension, hirsutism, and kidney damage. The doctors also recommend an experimental drug for acute GVHD—something known as "anti–TAC."* Encouraged by their reports of minimal risk and possible significant benefit, we agree to try it.

A consultant from the Department of Dermatology, Dr. Schneider, examines Liza and will perform a skin biopsy, required prior to the experimental therapy. He calls it a "punch" biopsy and likens the procedure to using a paper hole puncher. "Why is a biopsy necessary?" I ask. "No one doubts the diagnosis." Even as I ask, I know the answer. According to protocol, the diagnosis must be proven by biopsy in order to access the experimental anti–TAC.

"It's just one small piece of tissue," he says. "It will scar over and be scarcely noticeable. We'll take the biopsy at a spot that won't be that obvious." *Noticeable to whom, obvious to whom?* I wonder, steaming.

Liza appears to tolerate the IV infusion of anti–TAC without difficulty. Doctors come into her room to inspect her skin frequently, both those involved in her care on nineteen and many others from dermatology, to judge how red or raised or itchy or widespread is her rash, which varies remarkably throughout the day. Doctors often use the word "angry" to describe a rash, and at times, Liza's rash does look angry. I am still angry about the biopsy. What insidious process is under way beneath the surface? How great a problem will GVHD be for Liza? Are there weapons to defeat it?

＊　＊　＊

*Humanized anti-TAC, no longer experimental, was later marketed as daclizumab (Zenapax).

Molly in second grade shares her enthusiasm for math by making up problems and sending them to Liza so that she can have homework too. Liza treasures these gifts from her big sister, and when she tries to solve the problems, she often succeeds. Molly has made them appropriately simple. She also sends Liza a letter on Garfield stationery: *Lize, I have to tell you a secret. When Mommy is home, I miss Daddy. And when Daddy is home, I miss Mommy. But I miss you more than both of them together.*

Molly visits each weekend. Elena anticipates Molly's visits by having a game sterilized and ready to come into the room, and the girls play with each other with or without our participation. They also may watch a television show or a video. If Liza is feeling lousy, Lainie or I warn Molly, "Liza may not be much fun today." Molly tries to understand when Liza whines or pleads for silence, but she gets frustrated.

"Liza, we'll speak softly," we tell her, "but we aren't going to be completely silent. Molly won't be able to visit again until next weekend." And then Elena or I play a game with Molly while Liza rests or naps or watches TV.

The scrubbing and gowning protocol complicates things because Molly cannot go in and out of the room with ease, and she struggles to maintain the sterility of the environment. As she does not visit every day, and because she is only eight years old, it is harder for her to adapt her behavior.

"Daddy, why are you staring at me?"

"You are so adorable in this getup, Mol."

But later when I see her touch her hand to her face, "Molly, we need to go outside and clean up again."

"Daddy, we're in the middle of the show!" Liza protests.

"I know, but you'll have to tell us what we missed. Come on, Mol."

Chagrinned that she touched her face with her gloved hand, embarrassed and annoyed, Molly follows me out of the room.

"In the first days here, I had to regown at least three times a day, Molly," I assure her. "It was a pain in the neck! But while we're out here, we can stretch and shake our sillies out. We can blow our noses and go to the bathroom, too." She chuckles and goes to one bathroom while I go to the another, then we rescrub, regown, and go back in.

*   *   *

One day, after Liza has been on nineteen for six weeks, Cleveth tells us that she may need several half days off in the middle of the week to begin a nursing program. Elena talks with her about the logistical problems we will face when she is out: We don't want Liza to be in the hospital without someone she knows well, and yet Elena and I are also trying to keep up with our own patients. Some days later, having heard nothing more from Cleveth, I tell her that we respect her desire to further her education and move into nursing, but that not knowing if we can count on her disrupts us terribly. Cleveth becomes defensive, speaking so rapidly that I cannot understand many of her Jamaican-accented words. But I can tell she is angry and feels entitled to take this course and that she is trying to do as much as possible on weekends so as not to disrupt her schedule with us.

"You are the only other adult we feel safe leaving Liza with, Cleveth," I say. "And we want one of the three of us to be with her all the time if we can swing it. But if it gets to be too much for you, please tell us. I know it must be an enormous strain."

"I know, it's okay, I know," she replies.

"I need to ask you, Cleveth. Do you want to leave, to stop working for us?"

"No," she says with vigor, seeming surprised and shaking her head. "I wouldn't leave Liza now," she adds.

"I hope you know how grateful we are to have you with us, Cleveth. And we are worried about how hard this is for you. Elena and I have each other, but no one in your circle has met Liza, so how can they understand what this is really like, week after week?"

Her eyes fill with tears, and she seems unable to find any words. She accepts a hug from me. "I talk to my pastor about Liza." We agree to speak again next week. Despite her reassurances, Elena and I try to anticipate the possibility that we may need to be prepared to part with Cleveth.

On Monday, when she takes over for me at the hospital, Cleveth says, "I've decided to hold off on the nursing program for now. It's not the right time."

"Thank you, Cleveth." I know I should feel some guilt or responsibility for postponing her goals, but honestly, all I can feel is extreme relief for us, for Liza.

* * *

With her canny knack for anticipating needs before they materialize, Elena sent for sterilization two books we received from the head nurse. Lainie offers them to Liza now. Liza looks through one, a coloring book, and selects a few pages to color with the set of sterilized markers Elena also anticipated. Liza works intently, energetically, yet meticulously, careful to stay within the lines. Using bright pink, purple, and blue, she fills in the big bubble-block letters spelling out "I WILL GET WELL!"

The other item is a workbook from the Leukemia Society of America, and Liza takes to it enthusiastically. Under such evocative headings as "**When I first found out I was sick...**" it provides sample comments from other kids, arranged tactfully down the side of the page, leaving plenty of space for the reader to fill in their own ideas, reactions, and feelings. Because Liza can neither read nor write yet, Elena serves as secretary on the project. Sometimes I am with them; if not, Liza asks me to read what she has "written." On the first page, there is an illustration of a youth peeking from behind the page. He is saying, "Excuse me, but I think you've put me in the wrong book. I don't belong here." Liza chuckles. She returns to this page several times, shakes her head, and adds, sometimes with oomph, sometimes in a low-key voice, "You can say that again."

"**When I first found out I was sick....**" Elena reads the prompt and then the sample marginal comments. Liza listens and concurs that, yes, she felt just like Ellen and Kay and Michelle. Elena writes down Liza's response: *"I feel panicked and I don't understand. I was frightened. I am worried. I can't believe it. I think I'll wake up in the morning and it will be all gone and just like it was before I was sick. I guess I'll have to change my plans a little too. My plans didn't include getting sick. How did I get sick? And why did it happen? Why did it happen to me?"* Liza's comments float among past, present, and future. For now, she has had enough of the book.

Two days later, her interest is renewed and Elena reopens the book. "**The hospital...**" begins the next section. After hearing the quotes in the margin from the other children, Liza especially agrees with Rona, Ray, and David: *"I wish I would never have to smell that bathroom and hospital smell again. Sometimes I dream that I smell it and wake up thinking I'm back there again. I wish the floor were not dirty so I didn't have to always keep on socks or slippers. I was scared at first and real homesick. And I feel exactly the same because I had a tummyache for a while. I wish I never had to sleep there. I wish I never had to get needlesticks. I wish I never had to see nurses or doctors. I wish I never would get sick. I wish I never had to get sick. I thought the hospital was big and scary. It seemed like everyone was buzzing around, but at least they weren't too busy to answer my questions. The hospital is the most boring place I have ever been. Sometimes I feel like the doctors aren't being honest with me, when they take my parents outside the room to talk."*

Elena reads the next prompt: "**Side effects....**" Lizie certainly agrees with Michelle and Craig when she declares, *"I wish that I never had to have side effects. I guess the side effects are better than my illness getting worse. I wish I never had to lose my hair. It makes me really, really upset. It helped to talk to the doctors, especially Art Stevens and Lisa Mueller and Dr. Vlachos and Nancy Kernan. My mother would never let me write on myself with marker, but they do it for radiation, like with my tattoos."*

Then the heading "**My family....**": *"We are a lot closer now. We spend a lot more time together in our hearts. I like it when everyone treats me like I'm normal. I do show my feelings around my family. I get mad when I get sick—that's for sure. I wish my parents wouldn't nag at me to take my medicine."*

On the next page, "**What I am afraid of....**" Dan's one-word answer in the margin—"Dying"—threatens to overwhelm. Liza pauses. Then she says, *"I'm mostly just afraid of the dark. Sometimes it looks like there are monsters in the closet."*

Other pages refer to school and a social life that Liza has not experienced, so we put the workbook aside. The exercise has provided a structure for asking some of the big and obvious questions, especially with the help of comments from other children.

Elena brings in a blank notebook with a blue agate design on the shiny, hard cover, and she offers it to Liza. Liza wants to draw in it. She starts with a picture of a sailboat on water, with clouds and birds above. Next, she asks Elena to take dictation. Liza begins, "Once there was a little girl who had leukemia." Then she wants to do the writing, with Elena guiding her with spelling help. Using all capitals and plenty of space between letters, she writes her name, "L I Z A," something she regularly enjoys, then below, "I W I S H T H A T"— she stops mid-thought to draw a picture of a little girl on the opposite page. In the middle of her upper chest is a shape that stands for a dressing that covers her Broviac where it emerges. Despite several invitations from Elena to keep going, Liza puts the journal down, leaving it for the future.

*   *   *

In early February, the nurse collects an important blood specimen. Dr. Kernan tells us the results: 100 percent of the blood cells' DNA is from donor cells. This crucial information means that the transplant has engrafted successfully and that Liza's own marrow cells appear to have been vanquished. I recall Walter Cronkite's voice reporting from the early days of the space program: "We have liftoff."

A week later, Dr. Marks replaces Dr. Kernan as attending on the transplant unit. Reviewing Liza's progress, he tells us he may discharge her in a few days. The graft-versus-host disease waxes and wanes. A significant problem, it is neither going away nor getting much worse: With the combination of steroids and cyclosporine, it is contained. The hope is that Liza can be weaned from them in time without GVHD flaring again.

Regarding cleanliness, Megan, the head nurse, tells us that even though Liza now has more white cells than she has had in a year, our level of caution should be as it was before transplant—frequent handwashing, avoiding crowds, and staying away from certain fruits and vegetables. Then Elena overhears another mother talking about her preparations. Although they sound a bit fanatical, we decide to hire a housecleaner and a carpet cleaner to do as thorough a job as possible.

On one of my overnights with Liza, when I leave her room to take a morning bathroom-and-breakfast break, I see a nurse approach the room with a syringe of medicine. As he nears Liza's IV pole, I stop him.

"What are you doing?"

"I'm giving her five milligrams of IV Valium that the doctor ordered," he says. He seems to think that my surprise is due only to how quickly he responded to the order.

I interrupt him again. "Please check with the head nurse and with Liza's primary nurse. They are in the nursing station. I don't think Liza is meant to get this." He looks baffled. "Why would Liza get Valium?" I ask him. He goes to check and returns in a few minutes.

"It was a mix-up; it was meant for the patient in the next room. I'm sorry," he says.

A mix-up! Again! At least this nurse is direct and clear in his apology. Through my shock and dismay, I'm relieved that I happened to catch it. What if I hadn't noticed? Liza would have been put into a deep sleep from the Valium for hours, without anyone knowing why. What would the team have done in their alarm and confusion— tests, consultations? All of this happened in the hall just outside Liza's cubicle, and she is unaware. I want to linger in the bathroom, to shower, to shave, to scream. But I also don't want to stay away for long. Who knows what I am missing, what I've already missed?

Then, seemingly out of the blue, Dr. Marks says that he intends to send Liza home tomorrow. Startled, we check with Dr. Kernan, who comes by and assures us that discharging Liza is reasonable. Danger is everywhere. In the hospital and out.

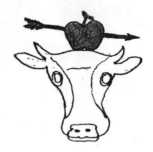

11—Home Again, Again
February–March 1996

As soon as we take off our shoes at home, our socks get wet. The carpet cleaners have just finished our bedrooms and hallway. When we all pull off our socks, we realize the novelty of being in the same room with uncovered skin. We couldn't even play "footsie" for the last fifty-odd days. Liza stands laughing in her bare feet on top of my bare feet. While she holds on to me, I dance around for a moment. It is exhilarating to see Liza reclaim her room, flopping onto her bed, touching her things, her toys, and smothering her menagerie of stuffed animals with hugs.

Molly arrives from school and we are reunited. Elena, Molly, and I all nuzzle and kiss Liza when she allows it. Elena and I unpack the large drawstring plastic sacks Memorial provided, in which we brought our belongings—mostly still sterilized—home. Molly helps by opening the sealed bags of games, toys, and stuffed animals that were waiting to enter Liza's hospital room. Liza and Molly play and run back and forth between the bedrooms, coaxing Elena and me to chase them.

In our new dedication to clean living, Elena and I require that the girls say goodbye to their three biggest stuffed animals. They have known about this for a while. With moans of lament, Molly and Liza hug Puffy goodbye, and then I lug the huge, blue stuffed animal Molly won six months ago at the Hershey Park ringtoss to the sidewalk. I come back for Barney, who many times accompanied Liza in and out of the hospital. Lastly, I haul away the elder statesman, Red Dinosaur, who arrived to celebrate Liza's reluctant renunciation of diapers some years ago. The house feels more spacious in their absence.

"By the time I took Red Dinosaur out, Barney and Puffy had already disappeared!" I report.

"How?" Molly wonders. "They couldn't even fit in a regular car."

"Maybe somebody had a pickup truck and just tossed them in the back," Elena suggests.

"I think they came alive and ran away," Liza offers, smiling.

✻   ✻   ✻

Before leaving the hospital, Dr. Kernan had introduced us to Megan Kushner, a different Megan from the head nurse on nineteen. She's the nurse practitioner who works with our group of BMT doctors. Megan emphasized that in case of any fever, we must call her immediately, "even if it is only two hours before a scheduled clinic appointment." Dr. Kernan recommends that we give Liza her own room to reduce her risk of infection. In classrooms and on buses full of kids every day, Molly can't help carrying germs home in abundance. So we sleep in a new configuration. Liza stays in the girls' room. To purify the air in her room, as in her hospital cubicle, we place on the floor a portable round HEPA filter, just larger than a hatbox. Elena and I give our room to Molly. Occupying our big bedroom and its big bed is a treat for her. For the first few nights, Elena and I sleep on the convertible sofa in our basement-level living room, until we realize that sleeping on the floor in Elena's home-adjoining office, also on the basement level, would give us a door we can close. We use a blanket, a sheet, and a foam pad that we can roll up; on mornings when Elena sees patients, we pile our bedroll more or less neatly in the downstairs hallway and quickly convert the room back into her workplace.

Steroids make Liza's face rounder. Cyclosporin brings her hairline down toward her brow; her proud forehead shrinks. Her hair darkens and thickens, her eyebrows become heavier and grow toward each other. There is a wisp of a mustache. But despite her changing body, she still feels pretty. "Pretty, Pretty Princess"—a game in which players adorn themselves with costume jewelry and tiara—continues to be one of her favorites. In dress-up play, she often dons necklaces, rings on every finger, clip-on earrings, and a touch of pink makeup for her cheeks. *What young man might be so lucky to become prince to this proud princess?* I wonder.

Liza's hands shake more and more often. Elena and I find this unsettling, and so does Liza. With tremulous hands, she can't draw as well as usual—the lines are not as smooth, and Liza asks us why she is shaking. We aren't sure. At the next appointment, we learn that tremor is a common side effect of both cyclosporine and another new medicine, nifedipine, used to control Liza's blood pressure—elevated by the cyclosporine. We hope that she will soon need less of the medications, but for now, she will have to tolerate the tremor. "At least we know the reason," says Elena. Liza grunts agreement.

Liza remains on a restricted diet. Her hypertension requires that she avoid salty food. Her suppressed immune system means she must also avoid food with high levels of bacteria, particularly the skin of uncooked fruits and vegetables. Even though the steroids artificially stoke her appetite, it is nevertheless good to see that it has returned. But the restrictions create tension. Before each clinic appointment, Liza registers her food questions for Elena or me to write down. Can she eat tomatoes yet? Gouda cheese? Apple skins? Pizza? Grapes? Ice pops from the ice-cream stand at the park? Baked chicken from the hospital cafeteria? Dr. Kernan always considers her questions one by one and answers, "Not yet, but soon." After a few weeks at home, Nancy sees Liza and gives the okay for the baked chicken. Liza adapts to her restriction from grapes and apple skin by fancying mangoes, melons, and citrus fruits that she can enjoy removed from their skin.

Liza's chief medical problem continues to be graft-versus-host disease, apparent in a shifting rash on her arms and legs, hands and feet, and sometimes on her torso—an itchy but bearable nuisance. The doctors want to reduce Liza's dosage of steroids so as to reduce their long-term ill effects. But whenever the dose is lowered, Liza's rash flares, wild and frightening, spreading even to her neck and face, until higher doses of steroids take hold again.

It's great to see Liza enjoying the simple pleasures of home—television, videos, books, coloring, painting, craft projects, cooking with Elena or Cleveth or me. She pores over her shelves of picture books or goes to the library and brings back a new stack. At home, she can dance or trot around without being tethered to an IV. Often she quietly plays make-believe, surrounding herself with her stuffed animals, a group dominated by her cows.

Her affection for cows began long before her leukemia. Two months after Liza turned three, Aunt Lisa gave her the first cow for Hanukkah. This was Daisy, a small black-and-white beanbag cow that preceded the Beanie Babies craze. Liza was immediately attracted to this "cowie" and formed a strong attachment to it. In a shrewd move, Elena bought four more Daisies when she saw them at the neighborhood ice-cream shop and squirreled them away so that we would have a ready solution in case something untoward—a rip or an indelible stain—befell the original or, heaven forbid, it got lost.

A few months later, looking in our closet for a piece of oak tag for an art project, Liza had discovered the hidden bag of reserve cows. "Look what I found!" she squealed.

"Those aren't for you, Liza," Elena replied, taking them back and hiding them anew. I think Liza understood that these cows—while not yet officially hers—would likely soon join her "cowllection." One by one, on special occasions or on none, each new Daisy did just that.

Like any avid collector, Liza groups her cows in a number of changing ways: by size, by color, by texture, by filling, by capacity to make noise. Though most are black and white, a few have different colors. Bessie enjoys special stature because of her rich, chestnut-brown hide. Another nameless bovine is adorned with a pair of devilish crimson horns and smart black and red shorts, but she isn't as compelling as Bessie. There is also a group of cow puppets. Two are spongy, meant for the bathtub; ten are finger puppets, a gift from Aunt Lisa during one of Liza's early hospital stays. Sometimes the finger puppets join the other puppet cows; at other times they stay with other tiny cows, like the litter of five miniature calves that can be stuffed into a large mommy cow. But despite all the varieties in her herd, Liza remains partial to her original Daisies and her one chestnut Bessie. Tenderly, she strokes the ears of each one, flattening them back. When the ears of one are just right, she moves on to the next.

Of late, Liza has begun to envisage a happy future as a farmer, but she does not want to wait until she is grown to get her own cow. After all, she wants "only a baby cowie. So when can we get one?" She sees no problem with raising a cow in our apartment. The real cow she imagines will be no more demanding than her bean-bag cows, only warmer and more responsive. Elena and I explain that a real cow might be difficult to care for in our home, but she remains undaunted. "If we need more room, couldn't we get a country house?" We answer that a country house sounds great and might be a possibility in the future. "When?" We tell Liza that she can have her cow when she is a teenager. By then, we figure, she'll have forgotten. For now, we appreciate the depth of her passion. The years ahead seem distant to Liza, but not impossibly distant. She accepts our plan.

* * *

"Do you really need the heat up this high?" I ask Elena in the day.

"Do you really need the window open this wide?" Elena asks me at night.

Now that tag-team life is over—at least for the time being—we struggle to share control of our environment. We know it's all trivial, but we can't help ourselves—we just need to vent some spleen. As we get ready to welcome Emily, Elena's dear friend from childhood and college, coming to visit from Chicago, we laugh at our rigidity; we declare that we are "putting it behind us," and we acknowledge the pressure of the past weeks and all our ongoing worries.

Emily, like Elena, is smart, steady, curious, open-minded, and openhearted. A woman with frizzy brown hair and intelligent dark eyes, her personality matches the generous span of her arms: She can enfold us and tolerate hearing about anything we are dealing with, no matter how upsetting. Leaning on her shoulders, hugging her, I feel my weariness, which I otherwise block out or keep in check. Based partly on her own encounters with serious medical problems, she knows how draining and frightening Liza's leukemia is. It has been exhausting. No wonder we've been snippy.

On her third day in town, Emily invites Molly to some one-on-one time. After a few suggestions, Emily realizes that Molly prefers playing active games to sitting and talking. "Molly, how about playing catch with me outside on the sidewalk?"

Molly eagerly agrees. Before leaving with Emily, Molly goes over to Liza, who sits in her pajamas at her favorite spot at the end of the sofa. "Bye," says Molly, politely. Grinning, Liza grabs Molly with her right arm, snaring her in a headlock. For a few moments, they are both chuckling. Then it becomes apparent that the headlock is going on for too long. The chuckles ebb and fade. Liza's face becomes steely. Molly appears distressed.

"Liiiize," she appeals, "please let go." Liza is silent. Louder, "Liiize, let go." I can tell Molly wants to pull away, to fight free of Liza, and she is strong enough to do so. But at the same time, she looks paralyzed with guilt at daring to step out and play catch, something Liza cannot do.

Tearful, Molly catches my eye and asks softly, "Will you help me?"

As I approach, Liza says angrily, "I don't want Molly to go outside!"

"What should I do?" Molly asks me quietly.

"We will help you," I assure her. Elena joins us as I sit in front of the sofa where Liza is still clutching Molly. I explain, "Liza, we understand that you're upset about it, but Molly is entitled to go outside."

Elena reminds Liza, "You had time with Emily yesterday. Why does it seem unfair to you?"

Defiantly, Liza maintains her clench, forcing us to intervene. I take hold of Liza's arm until she releases Molly, who is now in tears. Liza says loudly, *"You do not understand what this is like for me. Nobody understands what this is like for me. None of you even care what this is like for me!"*

I realize that, at some level, we cannot know how Liza experiences all that has happened, and all that is still happening, to her. Her face melts from angry to sad and heartsick. She begins to howl and sob. And we three with her—Elena, Molly, and I—cry too at the shock of hearing her fierce and unexpected protest. Elena and I encircle the girls in a hug.

"Tell us, Lizie, specifically what upsets you," Elena says. "We want to know."

front. Allowed to walk around more and more, she faced a lot of post-operative pain and discomfort. We consoled her with snuggles and ice pops.

Her eyes welled up as she asked, "Why do I get to get better?"

PART III

Heart to Heart

August–October 1996

And so you come face-to-face with the irrefutable lesson that many of us do not learn until much later, if at all: life is about loss. I know that sounds both fatalistic and pessimistic, but it is neither. Instead, it is honest and potentially freeing.

~ Leonard DeLorenzo

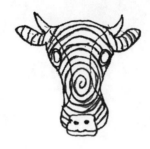

15—Questions

August 1996

Dr. Kernan guides us to the meeting room next to the nurses' station. She swiftly shoos some doctors and nurses out so we can have privacy. We sit in front of her. She talks with us for a long time. We learn the meaning of this relapse. "She will die from the leukemia. In months. Or weeks."

I hear Elena wailing. I scarcely hear my own sobs, but I feel myself shuddering. As if bobbing under water, there are moments when I am racked with sadness, aware only of my wife with me, and moments when I come up again for air, when I notice every movement and gesture, every word Nancy utters, and I can ask her to further clarify what she knows, what she thinks, and what her judgment can guide us in doing next. Then I'm under again, aware only of the agony next to me, inside me, my eyes burning, my face wet.

Elena's blessed face, her beautiful face, is my anchor. Her strong hands are in mine as we grip each other. For a minute, I am calm. Nancy's blue eyes are saddened, still bright, though less so. I notice her white hair—a sign of aging, of having lived. She is patient as the next wave comes. The howls I hear sound distant and horrible. They must be Elena's or mine. We set each other off repeatedly, sobs pulling sobs, my body bent over, my head almost on my knees.

Eventually, I am sitting up again, and Lainie is sitting up too. We are quieter, settled temporarily, as if high winds have died down. We can talk again and listen to the doctor.

We ask questions and hear every word of Nancy's answers, but our bawling, our passing my handkerchief between us and blowing our noses, our cascade of sobs muffle her words and interrupt her sentences. We need to ask again and hear the answers again. The doctor pulls no punches. Liza will die from leukemia, from this relapse. When? Impossible to say exactly how long. Nancy acknowledges that she herself feels devastated. Did she really say that it could be a matter of only weeks? I know she did. How long have we been sitting, talking, and crying in this room while Liza wonders where we are and why?

"We need to decide what to tell Liza," Nancy eventually says. "I suggest that I tell her. I can say that the sick white blood cells are back. How does that sound?" We agree that will be best. Shielding her is implausible, unthinkable.

"Then Liza can ask questions if she wishes. I will be available throughout the afternoon, and I'll check back in with her and you before I leave. And I'll come by again over the weekend. Liza can talk with me whenever she is ready. But we know she may just want to talk with the two of you."

"What do we do now? Is there anything to do before we leave the hospital?" I ask.

"Well, we need to stabilize Liza's pain. And you should see Dr. Steinherz."

"Why?" I ask, thinking, *Why bother?* Not clear what the oncologist who directed Liza's pre–BMT chemotherapy will have to offer.

"Not to cure, but to palliate," she explains. "Chemotherapy may give Liza more time. Maybe. There are reasons for and against. Talk to Peter. Let's see what his ideas are. He knows all the options."

"If we work with him, will you still be Liza's doctor?" I don't want to lose her.

"Peter may take over in a way, but I will stay involved. You can always reach me, and I will be following what happens."

"Good." We are glad she won't disappear. For now, we need to find the right medicines to stabilize Liza's pain. We need to see Dr. Steinherz. Then get home.

Elena and I, still holding hands, walk down the hall and into Liza's room. A minute later, Nancy comes in as promised. She is, as always, calm and alert, unruffled, but I hear sadness and dismay in her voice. She stands at the foot of the bed and tells Liza, "The bone marrow test from this morning shows that the leukemia cells, the sick white blood cells, have come back." After a short pause, she asks, "Any questions, Liza?"

Liza says nothing, but shakes her head no.

"The biopsy sites will be sore, I know, but are you in pain any- where else, Liza?"

Again, she shakes her head.

"I will leave you to have some time together, and I'll check back later."

After she has gone, Liza, at first pointedly, painfully, does not want to talk. But over the next hour, she begins to voice her emerging questions. She reads our faces and asks, "Are they sure?"

"Yes, Lizie."

She cries. We weep with her. "Maybe they made a mistake.... I'd let them do another bone marrow biopsy, because just in case they didn't get it right."

It is wrenching for me to leave, but it's Elena turn to stay with Liza, and I also want to be with Molly. Before going, when I have a moment with Elena, we decide to tell Molly the news when we are together at the hospital tomorrow morning.

That night, when Molly and I call them to say good night, Liza is muted, not inclined to talk about anything. It is hard for Molly. After the call, at bedtime, I read to Mol as we usually do, but I notice that she is distracted and I stop. We snuggle.

She cries, "I miss Mommy—and Lizie."

"It's hard when Lizie doesn't want to talk, isn't it?" She nods. "Liza's going to come home soon, and we're going to do all we can to keep her at home." This has always been true, but everything is dif- ferent now. Molly probably senses this, but she doesn't ask anything further.

A soft jingle of keys alerts us to my mother's arrival.

Mol and I call out, "Hi, Nanny, we're back here. We're coming!" We hug and kiss, so glad to see her again. All our eyes grow wet. She joins me in tucking Molly in for the night. Afterward, sitting quietly together, I tell her about our exchange with Dr. Kernan and what Liza has been told and our plan to tell Molly in the morning. Even as she asks how Elena and I are holding up, and even as I feel the comfort of her support, I recognize in her shoulders, her eyes, her sighs, how devastating all of this is for her as well—Liza's illness, the imminent loss of her granddaughter.

Later, while the girls are asleep, Elena calls again. Speaking quietly so as not to disturb Liza, she tells me of their conversation.

"Liza asked, 'Am I going to die from leukemia?'"

"I told her, 'Yes, Lizie.'"

"'How long will I live?'"

"'I don't know; I can't say.'"

"'Will I live to be a teenager?'"

"'I don't think so, Lizie.'"

"'I'll never get to have my cowie?'"

"'I don't think so, Lizie.'"

"Later in the night, she asked, 'I won't live to be a mommy, to have babies?'" Elena's tremulous voice breaks here, and she cries audibly.

"'No, Lizie.'"

Hearing this, I picture a wonderful mother holding a girl who would have become a wonderful mother herself.

"Throughout the night, Liza pressed me. 'I want you to die too. I want you to die with me.' And then she changed it: 'I want you to die right after me.' She revised again: 'I want you to die, and I don't want you to die.'"

Elena continues, "I responded, 'Part of me will die with you, and part of you will stay with me, in my heart, just as you will always have me in your heart.'

"Liza listened. She seemed comforted at first. But later, she repeated angrily, 'Mommy, I want you to die with me.'

"I told her, 'I would die instead of you, if I could.'

"'No. I wouldn't want that. I wouldn't want to live without you.'"

"You are amazing, Lainie," I say, "and so is she." Elena had been composed while telling me, but now she lets loose for a moment, and I cry with her. After a few minutes, she recoups. We rest curled up with each other, to the degree the telephone allows, and then we say good night.

* * *

On Saturday morning, Charlotte makes scrambled eggs just the way Liza likes them and brings them directly to the hospital. A bit later, after picking up a few items on the way to the hospital, Molly and I arrive. While Nanny keeps Liza company, Elena and I take Molly to another room. We tell Molly that the sick white blood cells have come back, that Liza has relapsed again, and that she will die from the illness.

Through tear-filled eyes, Molly asks, "How long will Lizie live?"

"We don't know exactly—we have been told that it will be weeks or months," I answer.

"Does that mean I'm not going to be a big sister anymore?" Elena and I embrace her and assure Molly, "You will always be Liza's big sister."

After a few minutes, she says she doesn't have any more questions now and wants to be with Lizie. We go back to Liza's room, and when Molly sees her sister, she says, "I'm sorry about the test results."

Liza murmurs a subdued, "Thank you, Molly."

Liza is in more pain. When she gets more medication, it knocks her out. Nanny, Elena, and I play cards with Molly. The girls have brief contacts during intervals when Liza is awake, but mostly she wants to be quiet. A friend comes to take Molly to lunch and to spend the rest of the day with her out of the hospital.

After a while together, my mother decides to head back to our house to rest. She asks me to walk her out. Before leaving the building, she hugs me and holds on tight, as if she would collapse if she let go. She sobs for a minute, and then, catching her breath again, she explains what happened when she arrived, sobbing again as she tells me:

"Nearing Liza's room, I overheard screaming and sobbing. From the hallway, I saw Liza sitting in Elena's arms. Liza cried, 'I don't want to die! I DO NOT want to die! I want to get to be a big girl like Molly! I want to grow up and get married like you and Daddy!' She seemed to gasp for breath, wailing and sobbing between sentences.

"Elena, crying with her, answered, 'I know, I know, Lizie, I know, I know.'

"After a few minutes, when it was quieter, I knocked and entered. Liza told me, 'Nanny, I'm going to die.'

"We three hugged and wept. Then Liza asked to see what I brought, and, grateful, she ate the eggs."

* * *

With Charlotte back at our apartment and Molly with our friend, Elena and I have some time with Liza and then, while she sleeps, with each other. As soon as she wakes, as if the question has been crystallizing, she asks, "Isn't there any medicine left to try? Maybe they'll come up with something new. I'd do anything to live." We tell her that we, too, would do anything for her to live.

In the afternoon, Dr. Kernan comes by. She asks Liza about her pain. Liza is quiet, disinclined to talk with her. We step into the hall to talk, and I ask, "Do you ever do a second bone marrow transplant? Is that worth considering?" She explains that this relapse is not the result of a failed transplant. The problem is that we failed to eradicate the leukemic cells, despite the powerful combination of maximal chemotherapy and total body irradiation. There is no reason to think that another effort would be more successful. Liza's leukemia cell type was "too mean." Nancy tells us that although she is not on call this weekend, she has come in today to be available to Liza and to us, but she acknowledges feeling exhausted. When we tell her some of Liza's questions and comments about her relapse and the idea of dying, Nancy's eyes well with tears.

* * *

Molly returns from her afternoon outing and has another quiet time with Liza. Elena and Molly go home for the evening. That night, Liza asks me some of the questions she asked Elena the previous night, as if needing to hear them answered again, needing to check if Elena and I see the situation similarly. Maybe she's looking for a discrepancy in which she can find some basis for doubting the grim news. Thank goodness I have the benefit of knowing of last night's talk with her mom.

"Am I going to die from my leukemia?"

"Yes, Lizie."

"How long will I live?"

"We don't know, Lizie." I imagine that our nebulous circumstance is excruciating for her—I know it is for me—but I cannot think of a way to make it less awful.

Pained, as if facing the unbearable, she adds, "How will I say goodbye to my cows?" I listen, sensing the depth of her affection—for her cows, and for us, the impossibility of saying goodbye to us.

Later, she is outraged. "I'm too young to die!"

"I completely agree."

"Molly will play with all my toys, and she will have more time with Cleveth." After a pause, she adds, more softly, "I've just gotten used to the world."

Every few minutes, Liza makes another comment, clearly working hard to understand her situation. "I want you to die too—with me!"

Her tone has an angry edge now, as if she wants someone else to suffer beside her. Liza the warrior wants to take someone down with her.

"This whole situation is disgusting!" I declare. "I know you don't want to die, and you don't want to die alone, Lizie." Before adding anything else, I see that she is thinking.

Again she asks, "How long will I live?"

"It must be so hard not to know how long you will have to live." I pledge, "We will make the best of each day we have."

She laments, "First the sickness took my body. Now it is taking my life."

A few minutes later, in a quiet aside, she says, "I've had such a short good life."

Later, when she is resting quietly, Liza's summation rolls around in my mind. She said it without emphasis, only understated certainty. How can she hold this view?

＊ ＊ ＊

In the morning, Elena returns while Molly stays home with Nanny. Dr. Fry, the attending on duty for the weekend, stops in and asks, "How are you doing, Liza?"

Liza is remote. Nonetheless, meaning well, Dr. Fry tries harder to engage her, albeit somewhat abruptly. "Are you scared of dying, Liza?"

Liza holds silent, so Dr. Fry presses on. "When my children are scared, like during a thunderstorm, we sit together on the bed and hold hands and sing songs. Maybe you should try that."

The doctor seems blind to our appalled reactions. Elena and I thank her for her suggestion and usher her out; we will call if we need anything. Later in the day, Elena bumps into Dr. Fry in the hallway, and trying to show sympathy, the doctor says that her own sister died at home surrounded by teddy bears. Dr. Fry seems to be saying that her earlier comments were based on experiences similar to ours. Elena asks, "How old was your sister?" She answers, "Forty-six."

* * *

On Monday morning, Elena, Liza, and I go to Dr. Steinherz's small office. He has spoken with Dr. Kernan. He says there are several chemotherapy agents that Liza has not received that we might try. With any of them, there would be side effects to consider. He will think about the pros and cons of the several medicines he feels might be useful and the sequence in which they might be tried. He will see us in the clinic next week, when he will make a specific suggestion. We explain that, now more than ever, we want to spare Liza having to stay in the hospital. We are eager to get her home later today. If Liza receives more chemotherapy, we want it on an outpatient basis or at home. We also discuss simplifying Liza's medical regimen. We review with him the many medicines Liza takes each day, and we pare them back to the essentials. No more light treatments for her total body rash. Liza has been listening quietly throughout, but when some of the medicines are stopped and with the agreement to stop PUVA—the light therapy—Liza raises her fists and smiles. Ironically, we realize that Liza's rash is looking better.

After the meeting with Dr. Steinherz, we leave the hospital and return home. When at rest, Liza's pain is bearable, but minor exertions such as walking around are often quite difficult. To remove the strain of going from place to place—whether from room to room or from home to someplace in the neighborhood—we've been advised for the first time to use a wheelchair.

In the afternoon, we head for the neighborhood children's clothing store, Lester's, to get Liza a new pair of shoes. Her feet are so sore and so disfigured by swelling that she cannot wear any of her old shoes, not even her recently acquired *Hunchback of Notre Dame*–inspired Esmeralda sneakers. We fiddle with the wheelchair, figuring out how to use the leg supports for Liza's puffy legs. We cushion her with pillows, one beneath her bottom and another under her legs. Once we get going down the street, I see that the unforgiving wheelchair has no shock absorption—it transmits every bump to Liza, so it is good that we padded her. I remember pushing her stroller when she was little. Now, a few years since she was last in a stroller, her illness has made her heavy, disfigured, bloated. But Liza's sense of humor is intact. Traveling as a small pack, surrounded by Elena, Molly, Nanny, and me, Liza jokes about being treated like royalty with her entourage.

The astounded salesman handles the situation with delicacy. He realizes that Velcro closures will be essential to enable Liza to get her shoes on and off with ease. Although he has no girls' sneakers in stock to fit her, he does find a pair of snazzy blue and white boys' sneakers that do the job well. In short order, we leave with Liza proudly wearing her new huge but comfortable sneakers.

Liza needs more and more morphine. When her pain is lessened, Liza, gripped by the narcotic, drowses, no matter where she is or what she is doing—even while eating or sitting on the toilet. As her head and torso drift fore or aft, she startles awake for a moment and then nods off again. She refuses to lie down and rest, insisting, "I'm not done!" whether eating or toileting. Because our time with her is limited, we don't want to spend it fighting with her. Nor do we want to leave her dozing at the table for hours between one meal and the next.

Our friends Aaron and his wife, Sarah, visit and offer their support. At one point, they sit together in the hallway, not far from where Liza sits at the table, somnolent, teetering, her eyes closed. I overhear them speaking softly. *"What are they doing? Is this life?"* Did Aaron and Sarah really say that, or am I projecting my own

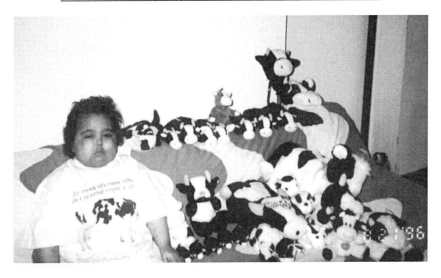

Liza, bloated after bone marrow transplant, shares the couch with a herd of cow friends. Her T-shirt reads "All I need to know about life I learned from a cow," August 21, 1996.

misgivings onto their barely audible murmurings? What kind of life are Elena and I trying to prolong? Will palliative chemotherapy allow Liza to continue in a morphine-dominated oblivion for a few more weeks? Are we giving Liza palliative treatment only because we cannot bear to let her go? Together Elena and I think about the possibility that it may be best to skip all palliative chemotherapy, though we understand that the doctors are unlikely to guide us in this direction; after all, they are doers wanting to help by taking action. We don't need to decide this minute. But it is unnerving to see Liza sedated, as if she is already gone.

Is she gone? For long spells, it seems as if she is, and then she brightens up again. Not knowing what to do, Molly steers clear, gravitating to Nanny Charlotte's side. Cleveth, despite her remarkable patience, is frazzled at times, especially when she tries to talk to Liza but gets no response. We all are missing Liza, hungering for her to return from her haze, wondering if she will.

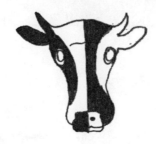

16—Did You Get That?

August 1996

At home, Liza asks again, "How long will I live?" When we acknowledge we don't know, she laments, "I wish I knew. It's hard not to know." She seizes on Dr. Steinherz's offer of more chemotherapy. Occasionally oddly cheerful, Liza says, "Maybe the medicine will cure me." Elena and I look at each other, unsure how to respond. Once, she adds, "Do you think it will?"

Put on the spot, I answer, "I didn't think that was what Dr. Steinherz was saying, but—"

"No, I think that's what he meant," Liza interrupts me.

I wonder if Cleveth spoke with Liza about the possibility of a miracle through God's intervention. We know she prays for Liza. This is tricky. Cleveth is as upset as the rest of us, and she leans on her religious beliefs to help her cope. Yet we'd rather she not talk with Liza about interventions by God.

Hearing Liza's comments about cure, Molly, too, becomes confused. One evening when I am reading to her before bed, she asks, "Is Lizie dying or not?" I assure her that she did understand what we told her—that Liza is dying. "Then why is she acting like she isn't?"

I admit that some of Liza's comments surprised me too, and I add, "Lizie may need to think there is still some hope for a cure, or she might actually be confused by some things that the different doctors have said. It's all so new that Liza's ideas and her moods may change quickly for a while." Molly's face relaxes, her easy smile returns.

Liza's hopeful moments alternate with episodes of foggy withdrawal, or sadness and dismay. When she appears optimistic and speaks of getting better, the rest of us must continue to live with the agony of knowing she is dying. Elena and I feel sapped. I am sure that Liza senses our uncertainty and bewilderment. Her fretfulness and anxiety return, showing themselves not so much in the old ways— with excessive wiping and washing, although they are still present— but with a free-floating nervousness that she cannot explain. When she is not sedated, she can be restless, fidgety, unlike her usual composed, focused self.

"Should we support her hope for a cure?" Elena asks me.

"It feels wrong to deceive her, and impractical. Beneath the surface, she knows. I think that's why she's anxious. And doesn't she count on us to be straight with her? Maybe she needs us to be clear and repeat that she's going to die."

"I think you're right, but that's excruciating," Elena's replies with a grimace.

I backpedal. "But I'm not sure. What if she really needs to be in denial? I don't want to take that away if she needs it."

"It seems so unlike her."

"I know, but we are in completely foreign territory."

"It's awful not to be on the same page with her."

"I know! I don't think we should be the ones to burst her bubble. Or to decide that she needs her bubble intact. Maybe we don't have to be the ones with the answers. Let's get Steinherz involved. His comments confused her in the first place."

We agree to let Dr. Steinherz bear the burden of delivering, or redelivering, the information about Liza's condition, the implications of her relapse, her prognosis. He was vague in his last meeting with us. And I know it's hard for most people—no matter their age—to take in upsetting news; often it needs to be repeated several times before it can be digested.

Elena and I tell Liza that Dr. Steinherz can best answer some of her difficult questions; we will write them out for her. Over the next day, she dictates some questions that I jot down.

I call him to explain that, as a result of the last meeting, Liza is anxious and confused. If she asks him direct questions, we want him to be clear and direct in answering her. Elena and I do not want the burden of giving Liza the medical information she's seeking. Dr. Steinherz says he understands our request. I have the impression that he is not used to speaking so directly with most of his child patients, and our request requires him to alter his usual style, but I am relieved to hear him agree readily.

In the interim, Liza does not stop asking questions. The night before our visit with Dr. Steinherz, she asks us to read the list of questions to her. She listens calmly. Elena and I have in mind to follow Liza's lead during the clinic visit. If at the last minute she doesn't want to ask him anything or seems to want him to be vague, we will respect that and will not insist that he address the accumulated questions today for our sake.

Dr. Steinherz joins us with his nurse practitioner, Rosemarie, and Ms. Manela, the social worker, and Dr. Thornley, the pain fellow. The seven of us sit in a circle of chairs in the well-lighted examining room. Liza sits between Elena and me.

Welcoming us, Dr. Steinherz says, "I know that you have some questions for me, Liza." I notice the way he says her name. There is kindness in it. He blends the sibilance of *s* in with the *z* because of his accent. We all wait to see what she will say.

Cautious and shy, Liza leans to Elena and whispers a question. Elena speaks for Liza, "How long until I die?"

He replies, "No one can answer that, Liza. No one has a crystal ball." I am frustrated by his answer, even though it is truthful. Is he waffling again?

Liza turns to me now, leans and whispers, "Daddy, you ask: Is there any cure for my sickness?"

I repeat for Liza, "Is there any cure for my sickness?"

"No." He speaks the hard word, not in a hard way, but definite.

From the quiet and shock of his certainty, Liza raises her voice softly—simultaneously plaintive and wanting to understand. "How can the leukemic cells cause me to die?"

"That's a very good question, Liza." He pauses as if thinking how to answer and then continues. "The leukemic cells take up all the space in the bone marrow, and then the healthy cells do not have any room left. And no one can live without making lots of healthy blood cells." He stops, waiting for her.

"Will I live to be seven?" This wasn't on the list.

"I don't think so, Liza."

"Will I live to be six?" I expect him to answer yes, as her birthday is just a little more than two months away, but he doesn't.

"I hope so, Liza. It is possible." Liza's lip quivers. I recoil. *Possible?* I exchange a glance with Elena. Her face mirrors the wince of horror I am feeling.

Liza, steady again, asks, "Is there any medicine at all that can help?"

"We don't have any medicine that will get rid of the leukemia for good. There are medicines that might help you to live a little longer, but they could also make you sicker. And you might need to come to the hospital to get transfusions or antibiotics. Do you understand?"

"Yes, I do." She takes a breath and tells him, "I want to try every medicine there is."

Dr. Steinherz appears surprised at this declaration. "Even though they might make you sicker?"

Liza's voice is no longer soft—it is forceful. She speaks slowly, as if teaching. "I know I may lose my hair again. I know I may get infections and need to come into the hospital. I know I may need transfusions. If I need to come into the hospital, I will do that. I will have as many transfusions as I need to have. I want to try every medicine there is. Did you get that?"

We six adults sit, astounded. "Yes, Liza," Dr. Steinherz responds. "I got it. That's fine—"

Liza interrupts him. "Then could you say it back to me, please?"

He halts, speechless for a moment before finding his voice again. "You want me to try every medicine there is to fight the leukemia, and to give you antibiotics if you need them, and to give you transfusions if you need them." Liza sits still, her back erect, looking at him and listening. With her eyes and with a subtle nod, she registers that he has understood her. "And that is what we will do. Okay? Did I get it?"

"Okay," she says.

The intensity lightens, and after a moment, Dr. Steinherz goes on. "Liza, although we don't know how long it will be, I can tell you that you are not dying yet. I will be able to tell you when the time is near. And it is not now." He heard me well when we spoke on the phone.

Liza listens keenly and nods firmly without speaking.

The exchange between Liza and the doctor appears to be over. I sense she is resting after exerting herself. Cautiously, Dr. Thornley asks if we have thought about hospice care, and Ms. Manela murmurs that she has had the same thought. They seem uneasy, concerned that Dr. Steinherz may respond unfavorably. Dr. Steinherz says he thinks looking into hospice care may be helpful, but he has no information to offer. Ms. Manela explains that right before our meeting, she made some calls and learned of two hospice programs that may work with children. She gives us the phone numbers to follow up on her initial effort.

Dr. Steinherz suggests a sequence of palliative chemotherapy for the next several weeks, starting with several doses in the hospital today when we break from this meeting. As we are about to do just that, Liza, who has been sitting quietly for the last few minutes, whispers to me that she wants to ask another question. I ask Dr. Steinherz if he can take one more question.

"Yes, Liza?"

"Can I see what the sick white blood cells look like?"

He thinks for a moment, and looking directly at her, he says, "I have a slide from your bone marrow that I can show you." I see a warmth in his eyes, a softening. Clearly, he is moved by his conversation with Liza. He leads Liza and Elena and me to a small laboratory area nearby. He fetches one of Liza's slides and sets it up under a two-headed microscope so they can view the slide simultaneously. He searches for a field with some exemplary white blood cells. Then he comes around the table to her side and gets those eyepieces in focus. He brings a better chair over, one without wheels, so that Liza can kneel on it to look in the microscope through the second head. At first she does not know what to do. He gives her a few moments to adjust to peering into the eyepieces. I hold her steady on the chair.

She asks, "Which are the sick white blood cells?" He continues to look through her eyepieces and uses a tiny pointer to identify a specific large cell at "twelve o'clock." I explain what that means, and Liza finds the cell, as well as some others like it. She lifts her head and sighs. "Did they have to be my favorite colors?" Elena and I take quick turns looking at the slide to see what Lizie has seen: Against a white background, amid many red blood cells, starting from its outer edge at the cell's membrane, the lymphocyte's cytoplasm stains deep purple and continues inward until it encircles the cell's large, round, deep blue nucleus.

Reflections in the Rearview Mirror

Change and Constancy

When my father-in-law, Sumner, was going to hear momentous medical news, he asked Elena and me to join him and Doris. Also, he had a pocket recorder—in the days before smartphones—with which to record the doctor's words. We were serving as witnesses, additional sets of ears to take in the information, as well as the tone, the spirit of optimism, the level of candor, the degree of clarity, and the quality of care, of personal investment. It is hard to capture all of that at once. At the time, I recall thinking Sumner quite kooky to want to record the meeting. Now I view it as shrewd. When our denying or distorting minds come into play, how valuable to have the data, the actual conversation, available to hear once more.

The imparting of important news can rarely be accomplished in one telling. It's wiser to think of it as a process requiring time and repetition. Liza's confusion was understandable, and we should not have been surprised by it. Elena and I appreciated Dr. Steinherz's compassion and willingness to go over it all again. In this way, he was a model.

✳   ✳   ✳

During a bird walk at Wave Hill, a nature preserve in the Bronx, I saw a stone engraved with the words of artist Robert Irwin: EVER PRESENT NEVER TWICE THE SAME. *This quote occurs to me as I think about the telling of this extraordinary meeting between Liza and Dr.*

Steinherz, or any other Lizie story that I've told before. No matter how much it is the same, even if I use the same words, it must be different also, because I am older, I am recalling it the next time, sharing it with someone else, in a different context.

My relationships with Elena, Molly, and Solomon never stand still. They can be trusted, and yet they do keep developing, changing. And I have, we all have, a relationship with Liza and with our memories of her. In ways impossible to calibrate, that relationship keeps changing too.

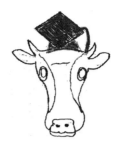

17—Supports

August 1996

While Liza rests in a day hospital bed receiving an IV infusion and watching a videotape, Elena and I take a few minutes with Dr. Steinherz. We thank him for his clarity and directness. He says he has never before had a conversation like that with a five-year-old. We ask him to explain his recommendations, and he describes his intention to give Liza chemotherapy that she can tolerate without major side effects. Though of course he cannot be sure, he hopes it will slow the leukemia and contribute to reducing her pain.

Later, Dr. Thornley, the pain doctor, comes by Liza's bedside. So far, Liza has needed extra morphine to control the pain, so the daily dose has been increasing. She aims to find the optimum dose of morphine at which Liza will be comfortable and less somnolent when her body has adjusted. I ask about using caffeine to promote wakefulness. She isn't familiar with such a strategy, but she will check with her colleagues.

As Liza drifts in and out of sedation, I feel myself foundering. Looking for added support, I search AOL's Personal Empowerment Network online. Under the area relating to children's health, I scan the categories and find "death of a child." I post a note on a bulletin board, briefly explaining that my daughter is dying. I ask for any parents who know what I am facing to reply. Selecting this category, writing this note, asking if there are others like me out there, I confront some of my disbelief, my desire to block out reality.

In this way, I "meet" a woman from Chicago whose son died a few weeks ago; her boy had been ill since early childhood from a viral infection that destroyed his kidneys. He lived for twelve years, thanks to two kidney transplants, before succumbing to an infection. The mother shares her grief. She writes well, densely, directly, no frills, no sentimentality, no evasion of her anger, sorrow, heartbreak. She lives with her husband and their surviving daughter, a girl a little younger than Molly, the boy's younger sibling. In this family of four, the constellation is similar to ours, except that their surviving child is the younger one. This woman had dealt with the possible loss of her son for years, virtually for all of his life; nonetheless, when he died, it felt to her as if it were without warning and perhaps avoidable.

I meet a woman from North Carolina whose son, high school aged, died half a year ago in an auto accident. She writes eloquently of her agony. Her experience is so utterly different because her son died suddenly, in the bloom of adolescence, a boy full of promise and talent, with a full social life, a wide circle of loving friends. She had no preparation at all for his death. She is struggling to keep her religious faith in the face of her anguish.

I meet a man from Maryland who has lost two sons. One died a few years ago at age six of leukemia. Like us, he is a psychiatrist. Like us, he first believed his son could be cured and then had to face the failure of treatment and his son's quick decline and death. His other son was older when he died, and I think it occurred some years before, but I can't retain the details, and I can hardly imagine his pain. He has one living child.

I meet a woman from Utah. Like us, she had two daughters three years apart. Her older daughter was close to Liza's age when she died of leukemia last month.

Each of these articulate people has had experiences somewhat different from ours, but we have an immediate bond in the form of the torture of losing a cherished child. Each writes from the heart. We wish to know and soothe one another, and these cyber friendships have an instant intensity and intimacy.

Many mornings, I leave printouts of the latest round of correspondence for Elena. She appreciates the vicarious contact, and though she is disinclined to join in communicating with strangers, she respects that it is an outlet for me. Energetically, she kindles an email correspondence with Emily, our close Chicago friend who witnessed Liza holding Molly in a headlock months ago. Just as in person, Emily's writing gives a tender and warm embrace. We email with some other friends, but Emily and my four strangers become our key, consistent confidants.

I find other grief-related sites on the Internet. I join some correspondence lists—one composed of patients, family members, and helpers in the cancer field and another called GriefNet, for people facing losses of various sorts. I find these diverting and somewhat useful. They help me feel less alone. Occasionally, people send amusing anecdotes and even some decent jokes. Once, I experiment with a chat room, but I find it unbearable.

Exploring hospice care, we meet with Ms. Ruskay at her home office across town on the West Side. A small woman in her early fifties, she ushers us into a high-ceilinged, spacious room painted a dusky dark pink. She smiles, calls us by our first names, and welcomes us to use hers, Shira. She asks us to tell her our story, and we pour it out. She is visibly moved and intently involved in our narrative. After most of an hour, she responds with a provocative declaration, almost chuckling as she says, "I don't think there's anything we can do for you." We realize the right and wrong of her comment. We are already taking good care of Liza and Molly and of each other. We have covered all our bases. She cannot prevent what is going to happen. But already she is providing something unique. She receives our story as no one else has—without flinching and with an appreciation of the richness and beauty in our painful, horrid experiences. We feel that this diminutive woman can hold us, can share and help us understand what is happening—in all its complexity and intensity—even if only by sitting with us, listening, and coming to know us. She also shows a capacity to appreciate the experiences of our children, our mothers, our extended family members—their needs and the impact of recent events on well-worn patterns.

As Shira learns about us, Lainie and I have a new experience of each other as well. We take turns telling Shira about our backgrounds, synthesizing what we have figured out about ourselves in our past psychotherapy. We are each smiling, saying, "I never knew that!" to one another, as we hear vignettes that capture our old wounds, as well as our strengths and accomplishments. I am moved to hear all that Elena understands and has mastered in coping with her sister's anorexia, her father's tyranny, and her mother's passivity. Similarly, Elena feels as if she is learning about me in greater depth as she listens to me tell Shira about my family saga of multigenerational strains between fathers and sons and fraternal rifts. Shira's way of listening to us leads Elena and me to feel closer. The sessions are long and intense, but we leave feeling recharged. For the hospice team, Shira embodies an embracing attitude. Although she never says these words, the message we receive is: *We are with you. Death, for us, is not a failure, but an essential part of life. We are familiar with facing death and the pain of letting go. We have no need to turn away. We are committed to helping you prepare for dying in any sphere—physical, emotional, spiritual. Our hearts are open to comfort you.*

Shira respects Liza's anger and helps us appreciate her fieriness that we find exasperating at times. While it is an enormous strain to be the object of Liza's rage, she has every reason to be irate. "What has happened and is happening to her is obscene," Shira sums up. Her choice of this word resonates with us. Our discussions renew both our patience and our creativity in helping Liza find outlets for her anger. Shira helps me recognize how often I turn away from confrontation with Liza to avoid dealing with her anger and my own. Shira's simple question, "What are you afraid could happen?" is particularly potent within the context of knowing that Liza is dying. I shed my hesitation quickly, and Elena and I reconsider what we do and do not want to confront.

We review a recent incident in which Liza woke in the middle of the night to go to the bathroom. Sitting on the toilet, teetering, she nodded off.

"Lizie, let me help you get back to bed," I suggested.

She refused, saying, "I still need to pee." This went back and forth a few times.

"After two more minutes, I'm going to carry you back to bed."

When I approached, she flailed combatively, insisting, "I'm not finished peeing!"

After I backed away, she nodded off a moment later. At one point, frustrated, ineffective, and exhausted myself, I lay down on the floor outside the bathroom and fell asleep too. It was lucky that Liza didn't topple to the floor in her somnolence. Reviewing the episode with Shira allows Elena and me to clarify our need to be firmer. We may need to be firmer generally, but specifically, we will limit Liza's time in the bathroom.

At home, we talk with Liza about our intention. She understands. Ordinarily, Liza works with us and whatever guidelines we impose. But given her fluctuating level of sedation, we cannot expect the usual degree of collaboration. A few days later, she appears to be in a tailspin, unable to leave the bathroom in the evening before supper. After a warning, I take the umpteenth piece of toilet paper from her hand. She lets loose, screaming, "Philip Nathaniel Lister, you are the worst father in the whole world! I'm never speaking to you again as long as I live! You have no heart! You don't care about me at all! You are the meanest, cruelest person on earth! I'm going to take off your pants and make you go outside with no pants on! You are just empty! You have no red! I wish you were dead. Just DIE! Everybody except me!"

Moments later, leaving the bathroom, she clutches me, sobbing. "Daddy, you know I didn't mean those things. It's just all too much for me, the sick white blood cells coming back again. And dying and all. Why me? I'm just too young to die. I love you."

I hold her as we sit down. "I love you too. I feel terribly angry and sad that you are dying. I know that the anger sometimes builds up and builds up until it explodes. It's okay." Her wrenching sobs subside and she catches her breath. I see how dying weighs on her. Of course, how could it not? Her distress sickens me. I am aghast, I am sad, and I fear her coming death. I don't want to lose her. I want to remember everything, her words, her affection, her pain. She gives me a huge, strong hug, and we go downstairs to join Elena and Molly. First, she snuggles up to Elena and says apologetically, "I couldn't stop wiping." Elena tells her she understands and welcomes Liza to the table.

A few days later, we have another skirmish. At our weekly clinic visit, Liza needs to use the bathroom before starting her chemotherapy infusion. I help her navigate to the bathroom with her IV pole. Unsolicited, she offers that she will try to let just a few wipes with the toilet paper be good enough. I leave to give her some privacy. Many minutes later, she is still in the bathroom. I knock and open the door to see her counting wipes in a rapid whisper with several mounds of folded toilet paper lined up to be used. "Oh, Lizie!" I utter in dismay. Poor, tortured girl, she feels both embarrassed and intruded upon. She fights me only a little when I insist that she stop wiping and come back to the bed, where the nurse is waiting for her. As we leave the bathroom, Liza looks at me and says, "Daddy, you may not be aware of this, but I love you."

Who is this wise child? Can she really be only five years old and select a phrase like "be aware of this"? Can she really be so attuned that even in the midst of our mutual exasperation she keeps me from giving in to despair?

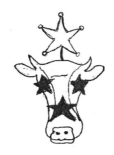

18—ALERT AGAIN
August–September 1996

As if sated by a good, long sleep, or stirred by a shift of season signaling the end of hibernation, Liza emerges from somnolence. In her sudden alertness, the morphine continues to control her pain fairly well. Most of the time, she says she feels "pretty good."

"She's back," I murmur to Elena. And for how long? For how long will we be able to enjoy this Liza? I feel this unspoken question inside, and I sense that Elena can almost hear my thought, sharing the uncertainty. My eyes fill with tears, grateful, excited tears. Let's enjoy all that we can now for as long as it lasts.

The wheelchair never suited Liza. Now she shuns it. We fold it up and put it away.

"Can we go to the park?" Liza asks.

Gladly, we take her. Liza rides her new blue bike with training wheels. She does not want to strap the black pouch with medication around her waist. So Elena and I take turns holding it and walking or trotting alongside. At one point, with Elena holding the pouch, Liza picks up speed as if declaring herself strong and powerful, and Elena has to race to keep up. Liza beams. Who would guess that the IV tube carries morphine to this radiant kid? Liza pauses to catch her breath. Then, without warning, she pushes off again, delighting in catching her mom unawares. They both laugh as Elena dashes to catch up—she cannot do otherwise or else the tubing would break or, worse, yank the Broviac out of Liza's chest. While I am sure Liza is aware, she is unworried, confident that we will avert danger. At the next rest, Elena passes the black pouch to me and Liza takes me for a run. Our girl is euphoric with the game she has invented. As if working a kite, we let out more IV tubing or pull it back as necessary. We are tethered to her, she to us.

A week later, I am in the same park with Liza when a life-sized sculpture of a cow appears on wheels, pushed or pulled by a tall, gregarious man I recognize from the neighborhood. Tastefully placed words on the side of the bovine advertise sumptuous barbecue at a nearby restaurant. I realize that I have seen him with the cow on the sidewalk, giving out menus and fliers for Brother Jimmy's, but this is the first time I've seen him in the park. He is giving rides to children. Four youngsters perch atop the cow comfortably as the man leads them in a long oval path, as if in an imaginary corral. More kids gather in hopes of getting a turn. I approach him and explain that Liza would love a turn, but because of the risk of infection, could he please give her a solo ride. He graciously agrees to do so, refusing any tip. As if letting him in on a private matter, Liza discloses, "Cows are my favorite animal." "A good choice!" he booms as a rejoinder. Round she goes, high atop the cow, amazed that this is really happening. A little anxious at being so high up, with the cow so slippery, she reaches for my hand to steady her as I walk beside her.

Liza enjoys the swings again. She loops the pouch around her shoulder, and Elena or I push her in a moderate arc, not as steep as she used to enjoy, but not timid, either. She enjoys cooling off with an ice pop, most often the red, white, and blue Turbo Rocket. By the end, Liza's face has become a big purple-blue smile. She sticks her tongue out merrily to provoke our shock and admiration.

At other times she chooses to sit on a park bench quietly. Wearing her sunglasses, her face impassive, her body round and swollen, she seems a small Buddha of indeterminate age. She says she feels "okay." She wants us to sit beside her, but she doesn't speak much. My questions lead nowhere. ("What are you thinking about, Lizie?" "Nothing much.") I wonder if she feels separate from the other children who are seemingly carefree, separate from her former self.

I imagine she is reckoning with some aspect of her illness and her ideas about dying. But maybe she's just resting.

* * *

Liza often asks me to read an Oz book to her while I administer massage. Either I hold the book in one hand and massage with the other, or I prop it open so I can massage with two. If I flag, or pause to rest, or come to the end of the routine, Liza pleads, "More mmuh, more mmuh!"

One night, late, Liza and I lumber upstairs to the master bedroom, where Elena is already sleeping. Liza perches herself on the bedside. I crouch behind her, and for a few moments, I use the massager we call the Wogglebug after an admired character from L. Frank Baum's Oz stories, a battery-operated, hand-sized, chartreuse beetle with four large protruding legs ending in purple rubber balls, and a fifth purple ball for a nose, which serves as an on-off switch—push the nose and the entire gadget vibrates powerfully. When I stop, I sit next to her on the floor. Liza grabs the Wogglebug and returns the favor to my shoulders. I melt. Seeing this, Liza puts down the Wogglebug and vigorously massages my neck, shoulders, and scalp for a few minutes. She jokes, "Daddy, take a deep breath in and let it out with a sigh."

Amid our laughter, Liza gets an idea. She carefully walks around the bed to Elena. She nuzzles and nudges her mother to shift her from lying on her side to lying on her stomach. Carefully, Liza climbs on her mom and sits astride her. She first applies the Wogglebug and then uses her hands to massage Elena's shoulders and neck and head, taking special pleasure in tousling Elena's luxuriant hair. Elena utters a groan of recognition and satisfaction with what the little masseuse is doing. Liza begins to murmur her own condensed version of the rap that has become familiar to her. "Take a deep breath in, and let it all out—either blow it all out or let it out with a sigh—and with each breath out, let the tensions of the day go, let the fussterations go, let the anger go, let the sadness go, breathe in courage, hope, and love, and get ready for the new day. Imagine a warm shower, then imagine a power shoot...." She speaks in a dear, soft, sweet singing voice. A few minutes later, she tucks Elena back in. Elena sends a kiss and murmurs, "Thank you, Lizie." Then Liza inches over to the other side of the bed, straddles my back and gives me the same treatment. I wonder what a "power shoot" looks like.

The next afternoon, I overhear Liza in a brief struggle with Cleveth at the end of her bed bath. Then I hear her asserting, "Cleveth, I think you're cranky because I'm dying." She gives Cleveth a little hug and then gives her a brief shoulder massage to restore her good humor. As she is saying goodbye for the evening, I see that Cleveth appears tense and upset. When I ask her what is the matter, she answers that Liza has just told her that she knows she will die soon, although she hopes to live until after her birthday. Cleveth finds it disturbing to hear Liza speak so bluntly about dying.

"She shouldn't think that way. She should hope for a miracle."

Elena and I review with Cleveth what the doctors have told Liza and how we talk with her—things we have discussed with Cleveth previously: that we continue to hope for many more good days and to enjoy every one, but that we are aware that Liza will soon die. We tell Cleveth that we respect her views, but that hers is a different approach from ours. We don't want to confuse Liza, and we don't want her to think that dying is a result of her failure to hope or pray for a miracle. Cleveth nods in understanding. She assures us that she only wants to comfort Liza, not to confuse or distress her.

I tell Elena that I yearn to eavesdrop and find out if Cleveth is continuing to try to sway Liza's thinking. Elena kids me about the appeal that I find in sleuthing, and then she admits that she wants to control what Cleveth says even more than I do. But we realize we cannot control what Cleveth says to Liza in the intimacy of their time together. Whatever the words, Cleveth's message to Liza is full of love. We also believe that whatever Cleveth says, Liza can handle it.

✻ ✻ ✻

One afternoon while Elena is exercising, I go with the girls to the nearby Woolworth's to pick up some household items and school supplies for September. Both girls love this store. (Four years ago here, while I looked for underwear, two-year-old Liza, down the aisle on the opposite side, found some cobalt-blue socks destined for me. "Daddy, you've got to get these. They're wonderful." Awed by the brightness of the blue and using the word "wonderful" for the first time as far as I knew, she easily convinced me that the socks were perfect indeed.) After loading up on paper and pencils, toiletries, and cleaning supplies, we are heading to the cashier when Molly finds some glittery nail polish.

"Lizie, look!" The two of them drool over the various colors.

"Daddy, can we get some of these?" Molly asks.

"Sure. How many are there?"

"There are a zillion!" Liza smiles.

"Let's get five," suggests Molly, going on to explain, "that way, we can do each finger a different color."

"Sounds good," I agree.

They each choose two and then collaborate on a fifth. As we near the cash register, Liza spots some earrings derived from her beloved *Hunchback of Notre Dame* Disney movie. With characteristic passion, she implores me, "Daddy, can I get these for Mommy?" When we get home, Liza asks me to get them out of the bag. She takes them to Lainie, telling her, "These are for your birthday, an early birthday present, because I know I might not be here."

"They're wonderful, Lizie!" declares Elena, whose birthday is in late November. She delights all of us by putting them on immediately, silly and superb, Esmeralda and Captain Phoebus snuggling happily ever after.

That evening, Molly and Liza return to a tradition they have often enjoyed before: Party Night. Held when the girls don't have to get up early the next day, it begins after being tucked in as they ordinarily would be with the usual bedtime routine. But as soon as that is over, they spring right out of bed to read stories—Molly serving as the reader—and play games. In tonight's episode, Molly acts as Liza's beautician. First, Molly applies mineral oil to Liza's head and works it into her hair, which is darker than it has ever been and short, between one and two inches. After Molly gently brushes and combs it, Liza looks chic with her glossy hair neatly parted on the side and her face a shiny glow. Since their party is sanctioned, they are happy for us to poke our heads in from time to time. Next, they set up small chairs on either side of their wicker hamper, which stands in as the manicurist's table. They take turns applying the new nail polish, each nail a different hue—light sparkly green, dark blue, light blue, sparkly purple, and a deep shade of pink.

* * *

In September, Molly will begin third grade. Were she well enough, Liza would enter kindergarten at the same school. Responding to my inquiry, the Board of Education tells me that a teacher can come to our home for Liza. I speak to the administrator in charge of the home-study program, a warm and savvy woman who collects Liza's pertinent data. We tell Liza, and she perks up and proudly announces the news to Molly: "I am going to school too!" Molly herself seems ambivalent about the start of the school year. She loves these last few days of summer, when she can sleep late, stay up later, watch some television, go shopping with Elena or Grandma Doris. I think she also needs this time with Liza.

A few days later, on Molly's first day of school, a friendly, talkative teacher named Cathy arrives at our apartment mid-morning. She wants to get a sense of Liza, but Liza is feeling physically uncomfortable and acts morose. In the face of Liza's dourness, the teacher becomes sweeter and chattier, trying hard to make a connection. But her efforts boomerang. She returns two days later with school materials. When she apparently overexplains one task, Liza blurts out, "I can do it myself." The teacher recoils, all the while talking, as if to explain why she had been explaining. A few minutes later, Liza pleads, "Can I have a minute of silence?" Although Elena, Cleveth, Molly, and I are used to navigating such requests, the teacher is taken aback. She seems offended and anxious, and in her anxiety, she cannot hold her tongue. While we are prepared to make the arrangement work with chatty Cathy, I call the supervisor with whom I had spoken originally to ask if another teacher is available who might be a better match. After listening to my description of our beginning, she agrees. She seems to have someone specific in mind.

A second teacher, Valerie, calls to plan a time to meet. I discuss Liza's manner and prepare her to anticipate that Liza might feel lousy and withdrawn. Valerie seems to quickly intuit Liza's style and needs, and when she arrives, she gives Liza some control over their meeting. She asks Liza to lead her to where they will work and to designate where each will sit. She gets out some work, shows it to Liza, and says she will sit quietly until Liza is done or wants help. She gives Liza an "ABC tablet"—a pad of coarse, recycled, off-white paper with blue lines indicating the size of capital letters and a dashed line in between to show the desired height of lowercase letters—to use for practicing handwriting.

Valerie immediately develops a good rapport with Liza, who responds well to Valerie's no-nonsense, matter-of-fact manner. Like the best doctors and nurses we have met, Valerie alertly observes Liza's state of mind and attunes herself to Liza with respect and sensitivity. She assigns work clearly, and she is patient if Liza seems unready for help or needs to rest during their time together. Soon Liza is telling Valerie about the books she loves and her desire to learn to read. Full of encouragement, Valerie starts with the sounds of the consonants and vowels in simple three-letter words, such as "cat," "hat," and "bat."

Liza is delighted when Elena finds a black faux-leather cushioned folder—the kind of thing given to doctors at symposia. It has a slot with a large ruled pad, a loop for a pencil, and a sleeve for loose papers. In the business-card-sized window, Elena identifies the owner: LIZA LISTER. Liza puts her penmanship tablet inside and chooses a snazzy homework pencil decorated with shiny stars and stripes to put in the loop.

Friends drop off food, come to visit. Sharone brings a glow-in-the-dark tic-tac-toe set and plays the game with Liza. Amid a lot of chuckling, they try to make the living room pitch-black so as to see the X's and O's glow. Eagerly, Liza shows Sharone her school folder and tells her about Valerie, her new teacher, adding, "I never had a chance to go back to school. Now, why bother? But I want to."

As she leaves, Sharone admits, "I thought I'd be visiting a sad family in a sad house, but it isn't; somehow you guys and Liza are all in good spirits, and this is a fun place to be!"

In contrast, Molly is fighting the doldrums, dragging herself to school, going through the motions, not at all like her usual self. Elena and I wonder how we can make things easier for her. We talk with her teacher and the school psychologist. We suggest that meeting with her classmates may be helpful—we can explain in an organized place and time what is happening to her little sister. That way, Molly will not have to carry the burden of her experience in private or the challenge of telling any friends she might want to know. Our idea would eliminate the risk, if she tells some people and not others, of rumors and inaccuracies. It would also spare Molly from having to answer questions kids may ask her, especially if at times she feels unable to talk about the situation.

With the agreement of the school psychologist and principal, we schedule a meeting with Molly's class. The school sends an advisory letter to parents. Dr. Thornley, our pain and palliative care doctor, will come as the expert spokesperson. She has become close to all of us during the six weeks since Liza last relapsed. Whenever we see Helena during clinic visits, she is generous with her time, loving in attitude, interested to understand what each of us is experiencing. In her direct, quiet manner, her practical orientation, and her earthiness, I imagine Helena might fit well in the farm life Liza has imagined, surrounded by cows, other animals, and children. She will tell the class about Liza's illness and prognosis and answer whatever questions arise. We will show the videotape made by famed *Peanuts* cartoonist Charles Schulz called *Why, Charlie Brown, Why?* Elena and I will not need to worry about anything, except being present for Molly. We can join in spontaneously if it seems useful.

We tell Liza about the plan one evening after dinner. We don't want Molly to feel that she has to keep the meeting secret from her sister. At first Liza thinks we are soliciting her opinion, and she makes her attitude clear: "I don't want anybody knowing about my business. It's private. No way!" We acknowledge her objection and tell her we regret upsetting her.

But I add, "What is happening to you is also happening to all of us."

"And it is important for us to help Molly's friends and teachers understand what is going on," Elena says.

"You're unfair!" Liza screams. "If you do this, it proves you don't understand me! Again, I don't get my way!" She cries and refuses to be consoled. I didn't foresee this explosion; I expected her to endorse our plan as wise and helpful for Molly. I feel furious with Liza for being so ornery and ashamed of being angry with her. She cries some more, howling, "Every minute of every day is hard for me!" When she catches her breath, she catalogs some of her privations: not being able to eat what she wants, having pain, having to die. After some time of our absorbing and containing her distress, her sense of being violated, Liza accepts our efforts to comfort her. We have a family hug. Afterward, Liza murmurs, "Sorry for screaming, Molly."

*   *   *

Molly and her class crowd into a cozy, informal auditorium with no chairs. The students sit in rows on each of the three carpeted tiers. Molly, in the top row, slinks toward a corner, nestled between two pals. Uncomfortable with all the attention, she is quiet.

At the bottom, Elena and I sit facing the students. Next to us, Helena leans against the stand that holds a video monitor. She is seven months pregnant and moves somewhat awkwardly. Her large brown eyes, made even bigger by broad, dark eyeglass frames, radiate gentleness. A native of Malta, Helena speaks with a British accent. After introducing herself and thanking the principal for setting up the meeting, she gets right to the point. She isn't given to drama, but hearing what she says jolts me. "We are here to talk about Molly's sister, Liza. She is five and a half. She has leukemia and she is dying. No further treatment can cure her." Of course, I know everything she just said. Nonetheless, I am staggered by hearing Helena speak with such unqualified certainty. Is it even more shocking for Molly to hear this? She listens, still and quiet.

Helena starts the video. Liza, Molly, Elena, and I found it helpful and comforting, watching it many times when Liza first became ill. Sometimes she watched it several times in a row. This short, simple, tasteful film begins in the fall of a school year when Linus's friend Janice develops a fever and many bruises. She is found to have leukemia and will have to miss a lot of school for treatment. We see her having many medical tests, including a bone marrow procedure. We see her receiving intravenous medicine in the hospital. We see that she loses her hair. Snoopy provides comic relief, first appearing as a friend of the schoolchildren trying to catch a ride on the bumper of the school bus. Later, he appears as a doctor in surgical garb, filching a donut from the hospital cafeteria.

The Charlie Brown signature piano music, here contemplative, plays in the background as Linus talks with Charlie Brown, voicing his sympathy for his sick friend's ordeal and his hope for her recovery. He is mystified. Why has this happened? Why to her? When Janice returns to school in the middle of the year wearing a baseball cap to cover her bald head, Linus defends her against a teasing bully. In the spring, Janice returns to school for good. Joyfully, she delivers the news of her recovery by removing her cap at the playground, showing a full head of hair.

When the film is over, our group faces the knowledge of Liza dying—despite receiving the best care and our best efforts to save her. Helena helps the children express their thoughts and fears. At first they have no questions for her, but then they acknowledge Liza's story by talking about the deaths of their grandparents and of beloved pets.

Someone asks, "When will Liza die?"

Helena says, "We can't say exactly, but probably a few weeks."

The children return to recalling their own experiences with illness and death. Almost everyone wants to participate. As our scheduled time dwindles, one girl brings the discussion to a standstill by asking, "What is Liza's life like now? How does she spend the day?"

The question snaps us back to ordinary life, the concrete reality of Liza, a child like any other. They want to know the situation in which Molly is living.

Elena and I describe Liza's favorite activities, television shows, and videos. We describe taking Liza to the park.

"Does she play soccer?" someone asks.

Elena explains, "She doesn't play rough-and-tumble games anymore because she doesn't have as much energy, and her body is swollen, so she's not as steady on her feet as before."

"I have some photos of Liza I can show you," I add, realizing I have a pocket album. It contains a hodgepodge of twenty-four snapshots, some from before Liza's illness and others during the two years since it began. Eagerly, the kids crowd around to see Liza, a real child, the sister of their chum. They look and look, trying to link the disparate images to one another and to the information we have given them. Liza's hair is variously long and fair, short and fair, short and

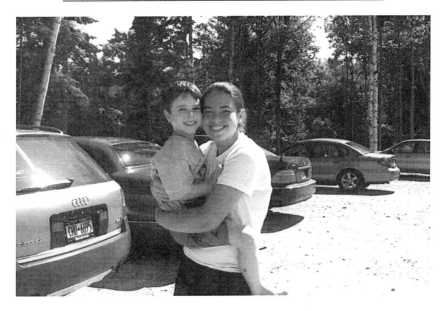

Molly, a high schooler, with her brother, Solomon, July 2003.

I held five-year-old Solomon in my arms as he looked at a photograph of two girls holding hands standing in the hallway, the same hallway, and at about the same spot, where I now stood.

"Who's that?" he asked.

"Can you tell?"

"Molly."

"Uh-huh."

"And who is this?" he asked, pointing at the smaller girl.

"I bet you know."

"Liza?"

"Uh-huh."

After studying the image for a moment, he asked, "How old is she here?"

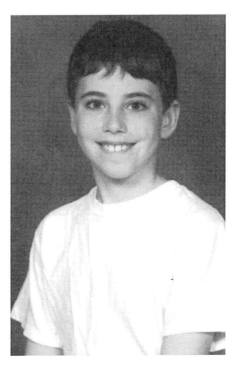

Sol in grade school, Fall 2007.

"Well, she wasn't sick yet, so she must be three."

"And how old is Molly?"

"Molly would be six."

"What if Liza lived to nine, how old would I be?"

"You'd be two."

"And Molly?"

"She'd be twelve, ten years older than you."

"I wish Liza had lived to nine and I'd have known her. And I could have touched her skin."

"She'd have loved you so much."

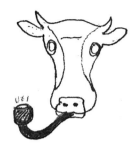

20—THE HAPPY SAD BIRTHDAY

October 1996

L iza will turn six. I am glad she will reach this milestone as she has
wanted, but then what? Will she focus on each new day "one day
at a time"? Will she try for another milestone—Thanksgiving? If not,
will she accept that her life is ending?

I take my anguish and fury to the gym and have a sweat-soaked
workout that's like one long scream. At the end of yoga class, quietly
lying on my back during relaxation, images of Liza in pain intrude.
My face is bathed in tears.

We plan a party for the Sunday afternoon before her birthday.
"My happy sad birthday," Liza calls it. She lists countless foods to
feature. She deletes coffee yogurt. "The last few times, it tasted too
strong, too coffee-ish." A moment later, she qualifies this with a shrug
and a giggle. "Too coffee-ish, I think, cuz I've never had any coffee
to drink." Liza makes the guest list of our closest family friends, but
they are all adults.

"What about kids?" I ask.

"Kalen and Johanna will come, right?" I nod—her New Hampshire cousins, aged fourteen and eleven, will be with us. "And Whitney?" I nod that Molly's friend, whom Liza enjoys very much, is
coming.

Liza still considers some of her classmates from nursery school two years ago to be her friends. It was not so strange to invite a few of those children to her fifth birthday party; Liza had enjoyed a visit with the class the prior spring. Now, however, an entire year has passed with no contact. Nevertheless, Liza says she likes three of the girls and wants to invite them.

"Okay, but don't be surprised if they say no," I gently warn her.

"I know, but it can't hurt to try, right?" Liza says, as if parroting what we often tell her. We call the three; to our surprise, two accept.

I phone Bruce, my brother-in-law in San Francisco, and ask him to reconsider Liza's wish to see her three California cousins—could they come for her birthday party? Elena asked her sister, Barb, several weeks ago. She said immediately that they could not come. Barb couldn't get any days off from work at that time; Ross is too young to fly. I think death frightens them.

"Please, Bruce. This is important. It's going to affect our families for a long time to come." At the end, I imagine asking, *Did you get that, Bruce?* The way Liza challenged Dr. Steinherz a few months ago.

"I'll talk to Barb," Bruce mumbles, "but I doubt the kids will be able to come." There is nothing more I can do. They are who they are.

* * *

The night before the party, Liza helps Elena make two rectangular sheet cakes. When they have cooled, mother and daughter apply the icing—chocolate to one cake, vanilla to the other. Then Liza adds designs with sprinkles, colored icing, red letters made of sugar, and candles. Elena guides Liza's hand in writing a large *Happy Birthday Liza* across each cake, as well as the number 6. Unlike the preparation for any other birthday we have known, the mood is sober, not giddy. Liza labors quietly for a long time over the second cake. She puts down an *L* and close around it, as if in orbit, the letters *E* (Elena), *M* (Molly), *C* (Cleveth), *N* (Nanny), and *P* (me).

On the day of the party, the phone rings early. In succession, the mothers of the two schoolgirls who accepted invitations to Liza's party call to convey their regrets. One has a cold. The other family must attend an unanticipated family function. Both sound to us like white lies. Liza is disappointed, but she brightens when she sees

Aunt Lisa, who arrives early. She has helped celebrate the birthdays of both girls since they were born. As always, in advance of other guests, she decorates the apartment with us. Tall as she is, she tapes up streamers easily, while the rest of us need a stepladder. She brings her guitar to lead singing "Happy Birthday" and any other requested songs.

Others arrive—Grandma Doris, Nanny Charlotte, Eric and Marcie and their children (Kalen and Johanna), our friends Meriamne, Sharone and Jeff, Penny and Bob, my college friends Chip and Ali, and Molly's friend Whitney. Despite her excitement, Liza is cranky as everyone arrives, comes in, and says hello to her and one another. Last in is Dr. Bobo, already in his clown costume: long floppy red shoes, baggy yellow pants held up with red suspenders over a bright yellow T-shirt; atop his head, a floppy newsboy-style cap worn aslant, with a multicolored oversized brim tilted up, and on his face, a slight bit of white makeup around his chin and cheeks, offset by a touch of rouge—background for a protruding, bulbous, red-tipped rubber nose. Over all the rest, he wears his white doctor's coat, with fake medical badge. Behind wire-rimmed spectacles, his kind eyes are smiling. He approaches Liza as if in slow motion, cautious and tactful. His presence cheers her.

The five children assemble at the table. After the lights are dimmed and candles lit, Elena and I bring out the cakes. We all sing "Happy Birthday." The singing is neither perfunctory nor casual, neither soft nor rowdy. It is tender. When Liza blows out the candles, we all cheer, perhaps a little too loudly. I wonder what wish she made.

Amid the buzz of merriment, slices of cake circulate (on *Hunchback of Notre Dame*–themed paper plates that Liza selected). Liza enjoys the first few bites, but quickly becomes "nausish." She has a little more cake anyway.

Dr. Bobo begins to entertain. Whatever we adults overhear amuses us as well. At first he jokes directly with Liza. Engaged, she laughs. As he continues, playing to some of the other kids, Liza quickly sours. It might be her stomach or just something about the fun, the ordinary pleasure. She pleads with Dr. Bobo, "Stop joking!" He stops speaking and shows his mastery of mime. But when he communicates in gesture, she protests, "Please, stop!" I suggest that he take the other children upstairs to the girls' bedroom. Liza agrees that this is a good idea. If she wants to do more with him, we can easily arrange it. Off go Dr. Bobo and the four kids.

Liza shuffles from the table over to the living room and stands by the sofa, holding a blue bowl in front of her chest should she need to throw up. She murmurs to the group, "Please speak softly." Her eyelids drift down until they're almost closed, and then they open, but she seems to be looking inward.

I whisper, "Do you want people to leave?"

"No, I want them to stay." Nanny offers to move over so Liza can sit, but she quietly says, "No thanks." She wants to keep standing because the nausea worsens when she sits. Sitting on the couches, chairs, and the floor, our close friends encircle us. Slowly, Liza sways side to side, back to front, sleepy and unsteady. Is she drifting away? Time now passes painfully slowly, yet not slowly enough. Eventually, the party ends. As people pass Liza, they wish her well with soft voices and then leave.

After a quick cleanup, Nanny, Molly, Elena, Liza, and I remain together. Liza remains distant, exhausted, very quiet, uncomfortable, nauseated. We eat a light supper while Liza remains on the couch, uninterested in joining us, half watching TV. After a while, she lies down on the couch and sleeps. She doesn't want to go upstairs, nor is there any reason to insist on it. Elena and Molly and Nanny retire early. The party has drained us all. I remain, sitting and, later, lying on the gray-carpeted floor, next to the sofa beside Liza, resting, intermittently dozing.

Sometimes I hold her hand or touch her, and I wonder whether she is dying now. At around 3:00 a.m., she awakes with a start, bouncing upright in distress and confusion. I take her hand firmly, reassuring her that I am right here. She squeezes back on my hand and then relaxes and lies down again. We continue to hold hands. A few minutes later, she murmurs, "Daddy, too tight." I loosen my grip.

I waken quickly on hearing Liza stir again at 6:30 a.m. As I sit up and look at her, I am jolted to see her sitting upright, appearing alert and refreshed. On this Columbus Day, Elena is working for a few hours in the morning. Molly is off from school. Liza suggests, "How about if we go to breakfast at the Green Kitchen?" Breakfasting at the corner diner is something we have done many times before. Molly is game. We get ourselves dressed and organized and walk the block and a half, glowing at this unanticipated treat.

Molly sits across the booth from Liza and me. In her customary way, Molly swings her feet. In a calm, clear manner, Liza says, "Molly, you kicked me."

"Sorry, Lizie."

"Can you not swing your legs like that?'

"Okay," Molly replies, but I see she is fuming.

George, the waiter we know well, rekindles our good cheer when he comes to take our order. "We'll share a couple of toasted bagels, and what kind of melon do you have today?" I ask.

"Cantaloupe."

He looks to the girls, who nod and smile and both say, "Cantaloupe, please."

When Molly unthinkingly swings her legs again, Liza, composed, asks pleasantly, "Molly, please stop swinging your legs."

"Why don't you slide down in the booth so you can swing your legs without hitting us," I say. Molly shifts, but sulks in earnest. I can scarcely reach her. The food comes. Now, with food in front of her, Liza's appetite vanishes. She nibbles without interest. Irritated, Molly eats quickly.

Home we go. Molly walks several yards ahead, as if tired of being yoked to her sister. Liza walks slowly, her black pouch with the morphine pump slung over her shoulder. "Molly's sure in a hurry," she says. As we round the corner, Liza asks, "Can we stop at the bakery?"

"Yes," I say, "we can do that."

Liza calls, "Molly, we're going to stop by Orwashers." Molly shows no interest. Speaking confidentially, Liza asks me, "Should I ask Molly to come with us?"

"I think Molly needs some time to cool off."

Liza nods. "Yeah. That's why I'm not asking her."

I let Molly into our building, and then Liza and I continue to Orwashers bread store. We ask for some fresh cinnamon raisin bread. While it is being sliced, Liza says, "Molly loves their corn sticks, right? Let's get her one." And we do.

As I help Liza up the steps to our home, she says, "I'm so glad we went out for breakfast and to the bakery."

"Me too," I say. Inside, we put our things down in the kitchen. Liza seems relieved to be back. Silently, she parks me by the sofa. Quietly, she goes to Molly and gets her attention. She walks down the hallway with her arm around her big sister's shoulder. I can't hear what Liza is saying, but I can tell she is comforting Molly, making it right.

They return to the living room a few minutes later. Liza suggests that Molly bring over a little chair and put it in front of the usual spot where Liza has taken a seat on the couch. She indicates that she wants Molly to have the chair face away so Molly will sit with her back to Liza. When Molly sits, her little sister offers, "Molly, I think you're upset about me, about my dying." And then she delivers a generous massage to Molly's shoulders and neck.

When she stops a few minutes later, with a sigh and chuckle at the exertion, Molly responds, "Lizie, that was the best massage I ever had!"

✤   ✤   ✤

The next day, on Liza's actual birthday, Molly is back in school after the three-day weekend. Liza has had to be up early as well, to get ready to go to the clinic. As Molly leaves for the school bus, Liza calls to her, "G'bye, Molly."

Sweetly, Molly replies, "Bye, Lizie."

Elena and I take Liza to the clinic. When her white blood cell count is measured, it is low, so she won't receive any chemotherapy today. Dr. Steinherz sees Liza and tells her that she will not have to stay in clinic today. He congratulates her on making it to her birthday. He encourages her to set her sights on another goal. Liza listens intently. Afterward, Elena and I speak briefly with him alone. He tells us that the regimen of chemotherapy he had in mind will be completed in another two weeks. He is unsure what to offer next. "There really is nothing." We know from a prior conversation that he would be willing to give a placebo, or we could decide to stop and tell Liza that the doctors have no more medicines to try. We will need to address this soon.

As we are leaving, we run into Dr. Kernan, who's been with us since she managed Liza's care during the bone marrow transplant. She murmurs to Elena and me, "It won't be long now." She has seen Liza's blood count. "The lymphocytes are increasing," she explains, meaning that the leukemic cells are taking over; the leukemia is getting out of control. We appreciate her frankness. She asks when the birthdays are, expresses relief that Liza has made it to hers and wonders if Liza will make it to Molly's. Nancy continues to be a straight shooter.

Later in the afternoon, when our friend Penny calls, Liza answers, and Penny wishes her happy birthday. Liza becomes chatty, telling her all about the Nickelodeon channel and her favorite shows. Then she tells Penny about her teacher, Valerie, who is teaching her to read. She declares, "With a little help from Mom and Dad, I did even more homework than Valerie assigned!" When Penny eventually speaks to Elena, she marvels at hearing Liza so articulate and happy after seeing her at her party two days ago unwell and glum.

Supper is a modest celebration of Liza's actual birthday—pizza and a small ice-cream cake. Liza appreciates both of these treats, though she eats only a little. She is nauseous much of the time. With the bigger celebration behind us, this one is anticlimactic. It is ironic that Liza is relaxed and in good spirits. We give her a LEGO kit. After dinner, Liza and Molly play with the cars Molly got her a few weeks ago. When Molly goes to get ready for bed, Elena helps Liza decipher the directions for putting the LEGO kit together. They work in unison, as they have on many similar projects in recent months.

That same birthday night, Liza and I finish *The Magic of Oz*, number thirteen in the series. In it, a character named Kiki Aru has the power to transform himself. When he is where there is no conventional food but lots of grass, he transforms himself into a cow, eats his fill of grass, and then transforms himself back. Liza chuckles at this. "Since you love cows so much," I ask, "would you ever want to transform yourself into the form of a cow?"

She thinks and then answers, "No."

I ask why, and she replies, "I don't know." She pauses. "I wouldn't want to eat grass." Another pause. "I like the way I am. I'd like it a little bit more if I wasn't sick, of course, and could find out about life."

I ask, "Do you have an idea what life is all about?"

She answers, "That's a mystery I'll never know." After a moment she asks, "Can we begin the next one now?"

"Of course, at least a few pages." And I crack open the fourteenth Oz book, *Glinda of Oz.*

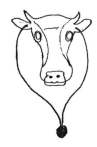

21—THE READER

October 1996

After dinner, Liza begins looking through the stack of newsletters from the Oz club. There are all manner of puzzles, games, and contests. A sprawling crossword puzzle on the back page of the June 1991 edition catches her eye. (Elena is a crossword puzzle maven, and Liza is inspired to give this one a try.) To our great pleasure, we find that we know the answers to many of the clues. I read them.

"Three across, 'Wind-up Man,' six letters."

"Must be Tik-Tok!" says Liza.

"Thirteen across, 'Royal Fox,' seven letters."

"Must be King Dox!" she declares.

"Twenty-one across, 'Always Lost,' twelve letters."

"Could it be Button Bright?" Liza proposes.

"Yes," I say, "it fits!"

Liza wants to write the letters in the boxes, a labor requiring great concentration. Slowly, carefully, erasing occasionally to stay within the grid of each box, she prints the first two answers. She poops out at the start of writing "Button Bright," but she wants me to leave it for her to complete later.

Much later in the night, she brings me back to the table to look at the same newsletter. She finishes writing Button Bright's name and then turns to the front of the issue. She wants me to help her read the cover story of *The Emerald City Mirror*, reported by Dorothy Gale,

"Formerly of Kansas, now Princess of Oz." I look with Liza at each word, sounding them out with her. She knows the consonant sounds and can start each word well. She knows many of the vowel sounds, too, but is confused by the variety of sounds each vowel represents. The longer words muddle her. To help her focus on one syllable at a time, I use my thumbs to cover the letters before and after each syllable, and then she gradually joins the syllables together. With repetition, she retains more and more, a mix of matching sounds to the letters and of memorization. By the time she gets the first few lines down, she has put in a lot of work. Excitement and pride now outweigh her fatigue. She wants to get upstairs and show Elena. After the usual bathroom marathon, we go up.

Liza crawls onto the bed. Gently, she nuzzles Elena awake. Elena asks Liza what she is doing. "There's something I want you to listen to, please." Liza moves over to stand on the floor next to where I am sitting on the bed. She stands upright, sturdy. She holds the newsletter with both hands while I illuminate the front-page story with a flashlight.

I strain to keep quiet and allow her to read until she signals me that she needs help, and then I whisper a clue, as if cuing an actor from the wings. Liza struggles to decode and remember the sounds that go with the words in front of her. "Dear ... Hon ... no ... ra ... ree.... Hon-o-rary.... S-si ... ti ... sens.... Citizens ... of.... Oz, ... Hi ... Dear—Honorary—Citizens—of—Oz, Hi!"

Liza takes a long pause, enjoying the cheering from Elena, and then continues doggedly: "All ... of ... us ... here ... in ... the.... Em ... er ... uld.... Emmeruld.... Emerald.... S-si ... tee.... City.... Em'rald City ... (es ... pesh ... ill ... lee ... espesheeullee ... especially ... thuuh.... Wizz ... ard ... the—Wizard ... and ... the.... Wah ... gull ... bug.... Wog ... gle ... bug ... the—Wogglebug) ... have ... been ... wor ... king ... work-ing ... day ... and ... night ... or ... gan ... iz ... ing ... or-gan-i-zing ... the Roy ... all.... Roy-al.... Culub.... Club ... of Oz." She is gleeful as she finishes her mini-marathon. Elena and I applaud.

Liza says, "I'll surprise Cleveth by reading this to her tomorrow."

"Later today, actually," I say, and she chuckles.

When Cleveth arrives in the early afternoon, Liza and Valerie are beginning their tutorial. As soon as Liza sees Cleveth, she interrupts her schoolwork, takes Cleveth's hand, and leads her down the hallway. Asking Cleveth to "Wait here," she fetches the Oz newsletter and walks back to Cleveth. Liza positions Cleveth and then steps right in front of her left leg, so that Cleveth, with her yellow dress almost touching Liza's back, is looking over Liza's right shoulder.

Standing under a high-hat light fixture that provides a spotlight, Liza holds the paper in front of her. (She has agreed to let me videotape her.) With all our attention focused on her, Liza begins her repeat performance. This time there is more difficulty, more shifts back to the beginning. With good intention, Cleveth offers help quickly. Liza recoils, complaining, "Don't tell me unless I ask you, Cleveth!" Liza holds herself together and stumbles through the sentence. We show our appreciation. Although the moment falls short of last night's magic, it is impressive nevertheless.

Not only have Dr. Kernan's comments alerted us that these are Liza's last days, we also see it in Liza. When sleeping, she is densely asleep, almost gone. When we try to rouse her in late mornings or early afternoons, she doesn't respond until we shout and shake her persistently. Sometimes even then we cannot reach her except for a murmur, and we try again later. When she is awake, she is constantly nauseated, has no appetite. To control her pain, she requires extra doses of morphine again. She looks weary and moves more slowly, always carrying a blue plastic bowl in case she spits up. She still enjoys spells of playing with toys, watching TV, doing her homework, listening to stories—all of her usual activities—but she tires quickly and rests limply.

At home with Liza, Elena is full of energy and affirmation, a model for me. Liza inspires us both to do all we can. When Cleveth is with Liza, Lainie and I go outside for a walk and share our observations of Liza's decline—her physical unsteadiness and weakness, her dulled glassy eyes, her swollenness, her moments of withdrawal, her surprising but brief energetic dances. By phone, we ask Dr. Thornley which medications to give Liza and at what dosages and intervals. We discuss with one another how Molly is doing and think about how we can best take care of her. We do not sink into sadness because there is still work to do. We each have our tearful breakdowns, usually with each other, and then we regroup, engaged with the work at hand.

Often we burst into laughter, sick laughter, at hearing a gruesome bit of news that in the past might have repelled us. Now we think, *Anything can happen to anyone. Security is a joke!* I try with humor to immunize us against the pain ahead with images of calamity that could strike either one of us, or another loved one, or our home up in smoke. Why not? We think of former silly concerns— matching shoes to an outfit, matching an outfit to an occasion. "Maybe you worried about that; I don't believe I ever did," I say, causing Elena's jaw to drop, her eyes to sparkle.

❉ ❉ ❉

There is some business to attend to. We know we want Liza to be cremated, as Leonard and Sumner were. What we will do with the ashes (the "cremains"), we needn't decide now. We want her body autopsied so as to understand all we possibly can about her disease, and we want to donate any part of Liza's body that can be of use to medical science. Elena calls Dr. Kernan, who explains that studying Liza's thymus (a small gland in the upper chest important to the immune system, particularly in the maturation of T lymphocytes) could be of use, but not the rest of her body. An autopsy can be done at Memorial and the thymus gland removed for study. Elena learns what steps we need to take.

We need to find a funeral home to transport Liza's body to the hospital, then to a mortuary for a service, and then to a crematorium. Elena gets some recommendations and follows up with phone calls. We meet with Marty Kasdan, the funeral director at Riverside Memorial Chapel on Manhattan's West Side. He gives us the same feeling we had when we met Shira: compassion, respect, comprehension of our circumstances, the capacity to contain us, to deal with us without armor. We fill out preliminary papers, see two chapels and several rooms in which we can hold a service for Liza, and are told about what the procedures will be when the time comes.

❉ ❉ ❉

Liza seems to be going to the bathroom much less, sometimes only twice a day or even once. Can this be so? Are her bodily functions slowing? Is she holding back, to avoid all that she puts herself through when she's in the bathroom? When she is on the toilet, I busy myself with emailing my pen pals. The compassionate notes I receive are a solace, often bringing me to tears. After a while, I give Liza a warning call and then go to see if she has been able to manage. I find her giving up on any more wiping, but Liza looks drained. I emulate my wise wife and say, "If it's too much for you—all the struggle and pain and nausea—we understand. We will be okay."

She listens and says quietly, "I don't want to die."

I tell her, "I don't want you to die either."

A moment later: "Why me." She has said these words before, but today they strike me neither as question nor protest, not so pained as before, but more as resignation. I nod in some kind of inarticulate agreement. Liza says, "I've been thinking about heaven some more. I hope I see Poppy Leonard and Grandpa Sumner."

I say, "If there is a heaven, they might be with other people they loved; you might meet them, and I bet they would surely love you too." Consciously, I am trying to ease her anxiety about being alone, but I am finding comfort myself in a notion of human interconnection, as if Liza's spirit could join a sea of spirits of those who have gone before her.

That night, after watching her shows, Liza slips off my lap and begins rummaging through her special objects. In a change from her routine, she goes to the cabinet where we keep her small collection of kid-sized musical instruments—an accordion, a saxophone, a guitar, a pennywhistle, a xylophone, a drum. Liza loved to play with them before she became ill. But for the last two years, she has shunned them—sounds have too easily irritated her. I am surprised to see her return to them now. She selects her harmonica. She sits and plays it patiently, sweetly, softly, studiously, as if she is working out something important. At length I ask her, "What is this song you are playing, Lizie?"

She explains, "Talking about heaven made me think of a song in my mind. It has to do with the heart." She plays some more and then agrees when I suggest we go upstairs. In the master bedroom, she sits on the floor at the end of the bed. She plays a few long, soft notes and then whispers, "Do you think playing will disturb Mommy?"

"Not a bit." She plays on for another twenty-five minutes.

For the next three nights, she repeats this musical interlude before going upstairs to bed. One evening, she experiments with adding each of her other instruments to her composition, playing each earnestly, sometimes going back to the harmonica for a few notes before moving on to another instrument. Then she puts all the instruments away, reserving only the harmonica, which she plays with absorption. From now on, it travels with her upstairs at bedtime and downstairs when she wakes, along with Liza's other treasured objects.

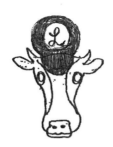

22—Molly's Birthday

October 1996

The next day, Friday, October 25, is Molly's ninth birthday. We plan to go to dinner—the immediate family and Nanny—to Serendipity 3, a restaurant twenty blocks from our house. We celebrated Molly's graduation from kindergarten there. Molly, Liza, and I all loved their signature drink, "frozen hot chocolate," a dessert extravaganza served in a huge goblet and large enough to be a meal in itself. We discuss ordering it again. But as evening approaches, Liza becomes increasingly uncomfortable. Her pain and nausea require extra medication, and she has no appetite. She has trouble mobilizing to get dressed. Elena and I decide that I should go ahead with Molly and Nanny to the restaurant.

With effort, Elena and Liza get out of the house and into a taxi. On the way, Liza reflects on her effort. She says to Elena, "It might make me upset, it might make me uncomfortable, but I'm not going to let that stop me. Molly's birthday is important for me too because Molly is my big sister. We like a lot of the same things. And we look alike. She has gotten me presents. And she reads to me. And she teaches me things."

By the time they get to our table, we are finishing dinner. Liza feels too nauseated to eat anyway. She holds her blue bowl in front of her chest in the restaurant. Even so, she is beaming, albeit faintly. Though she looks bloated and pale and feels awful, she is glad to be part of the birthday event and joins in stoutly singing "Happy Birthday" as the waiter brings our desserts. Nanny gasps on seeing the chocolate excess for the first time; the rest of us laugh. Liza has the first little sip of my frozen hot chocolate, but no more. She remains on Elena's lap staying as still as she can, following the conversation some of the time, not saying much.

Back home, Elena and I discuss the bigger party we have planned for midday tomorrow. Molly's friends will join her at Leisure Time Bowling at the Port Authority Bus Terminal. After tonight's effort and seeing how weak, uncomfortable, and remote Liza seems now, it is hard to imagine her getting going again in fifteen hours. If Liza cannot go there, what should we do? We don't want Molly to lose her party at the last minute. We call Aunt Lisa and Sharone and Penny and ask them to help host the party by arriving early and shepherding the twenty-odd kids to their designated bowling lanes, to tables for pizza, and back to the lanes for a final game. They agree, and if we need to cancel at the last minute, they will help with that, too. As I did tonight, I will go ahead with Molly and Nanny; Elena and Liza will join us if they can.

We can see that Liza is declining, but Elena and I still have a lot of questions. I call Dr. Thornley and ask, "Knowing this is not an exact science, but drawing on your experience, how long is Liza's dying likely to take? Will she make it until tomorrow night?"

"Almost certainly" is her educated guess. Elena and I realize that, despite our discussion with Shira, we continue to hope that we will all be together with Liza when she dies.

At the moment, Liza is sleeping while sitting in her favorite spot on the gray sofa. None of us want to leave her. Elena sleeps on the small, brown couch at a right angle to the gray one. Molly sleeps with a pillow on the floor nearer the dining room. I stay up writing email and watching over the three of them, until, finally, I lie on the floor in front of Liza and sleep too.

Late the next morning, Molly, Nanny, and I head to the bowling alley. Liza says goodbye, adding that she intends to join us. We all want to be at Molly's party, but I am in a daze, preoccupied, wondering what is happening with Liza at home. The parents of Molly's schoolmates don't know how to help. Thank goodness for Sharone,

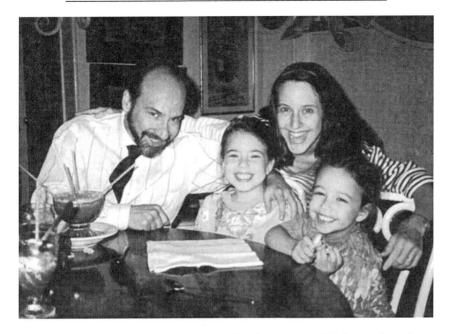

We celebrate Molly's graduation from kindergarten (with frozen hot chocolate), June 1994.

Penny, and Lisa. They prop me up, joke with me about the silliness of seeing the kids hoisting bowling balls too heavy for them, and offer plenty of hugs. I have some fun with Molly's friends and help a few of them with the bowling—although with bumpers in the lanes, everyone knocks down a few pins.

Midway through the party, my beeper goes off; I am being paged to a phone number I don't recognize. Over the din of the crashing bowling pins and the too-loud background pop music, I make out Elena's voice. She and Liza can't make it to the party. Liza just wants to sit still on Elena's lap. But a problem has come up. A mailman buzzed to deliver a package. Elena, with Liza in her arms, went to retrieve the package from the building foyer, and as she did so, the door to our apartment swung locked behind her. In her nightgown and holding Liza in pajamas, Elena buzzed our neighbor and paged me from his apartment. They will stay there until someone comes home. I want to go, but I feel it best to stay with Molly. Penny takes the keys. I call home a little later and Elena answers. We laugh about the incident, Murphy's Law. Relieved, I note, "At least Liza was with you! Imagine her inside, downstairs alone wondering what happened to you."

Getting off the phone, I try to calm down and enjoy the spirit of the party. After pizza and a final round of bowling, children and parents reconvene at our table. An ice-cream birthday cake appears, and we all sing "Happy Birthday." Molly blows out her candles, a happy task she does easily, in stark contrast to the effort Liza mustered two weeks ago. Molly is being a terrific sport, and she actually is having a good time.

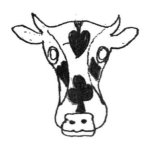

23—Time

When we get home, Elena says that Liza has been glued to her lap for almost the entire time. Foggy, Liza has no appetite. She only sips water.

I call Helena Thornley, and she tells me how much extra morphine to give Liza, how much Valium, how much antiemetic. Helena plans to visit us in several hours, and she arrives mid-evening. She comes to the living room to observe and speak with Liza. "Hi, Lizie. It's Hellie. How are you doing, love?"

With terse replies and nods, Liza answers her questions and tells her about her pain, nausea, and difficulty breathing. Taking what she needs from the boxes of medical supplies that line our dining room, Helena gives her more medicine, then moves across the room to wait and observe.

Liza asks, "Can we turn on the TV to see *I Love Lucy*?" We do, but after a few minutes, she wants it off. A few minutes later, she asks, "Can we listen to my lullaby tape?" Nanny gets it from upstairs, where it has always been for Liza to listen to at bedtime. For the first time, we play the tape downstairs. Liza seems to enjoy it, if only wispily. When the second song ends, she asks that it be turned off. She asks for quiet. She asks that we turn down the lights. Nanny withdraws to Elena's office. Molly goes to her room. It grows late.

When Elena needs to go to the bathroom, Liza asks me to come beside her. She is standing next to the sofa, waiting for Elena to return to sit under her. I kneel beside Liza. Nestling, she melts into

255

me, melting me. She holds me tenderly. I return her embrace, careful not to squeeze too hard. After Elena resumes her station, Liza's breathing becomes more ragged. She retches without bringing anything up. Helena gives her more medicine.

I see Helena search for and find a piece of paper and a pen. Intuiting that she wants to communicate with me unobtrusively, I get up from beside Elena and Liza. Reaching the dining room table, I see that she has begun a note to me with the words *She is still fighting....* Helena says to me quietly, "Liza is fighting the medicine. I've never seen anything like this, to give this much narcotic with so little effect. You need to tell her that it's okay to let go."

I understand immediately that this is so. Liza's death is at hand. I also have this angry thought in a corner of my mind: *How the hell do you know?* But I know too.

I kneel in front of Liza, who is still perched on Elena's lap. Liza has a request. "Daddy, if you go out anywhere, please leave your hanky with me." She holds the recently borrowed, dark green hanky in her hand.

"You don't need to worry about my hanky, Lizie. I'm happy for you to have it."

"Mommy, Daddy's nervous," Liza notes astutely.

Softly, Elena says, "It looks like he has something important to say." Elena has noticed that I conferred with Helena. I think Elena knows what I am about to say.

I continue, choking up a little, "But also, I'm not going anywhere. I'm staying right here with you and Mommy. Do you want to know why?"

"Uh-huh."

"Hearing you play the lullaby tape and seeing you on Mommy's lap like this, I realize it is time, time to let go."

Liza replies, reaching to the heart of the matter, "It's not the tape, Daddy. It's me."

"Yes, it's you. The time of dying is here."

Liza protests, "But Dr. Steinherz didn't call!"

Helena has been sitting near enough to hear us. Without a moment's delay, she comes over to Liza and offers a graceful lie. "Dr. Steinherz sent me in his place to tell you in person."

Liza winces. Her mouth quivers as she registers the imminence of death. Elena is holding her gently, steadily, bracing her, comforting her. Looking past Lizie, I see my wife's weeping eyes. She looks back at me. I feel her agony and her love.

But then Liza girds herself and says, "I need to see Molly and Cleveth."

Helena finds my mother and asks her to go upstairs to get Molly, who has conked out in her bedroom. Cleveth is in Brooklyn at a family birthday gathering, celebrating her own October birthday and those of three members of her extended family. I call and get Cleveth on the phone while bleary-eyed Molly comes down and stands in front of Liza. Poised and valiant, Liza says, "Molly, we think it's time I'm going to die. I just want you to know I really love you." Molly appears overwhelmed, almost staggered. She takes a few small steps and stands nearby.

Liza takes the phone from me. "Cleveth, we think it's time I'm going to die. I just want you to know I love you." While Liza listens, I imagine that Cleveth, shaken, is telling Liza that she wants to visit, but that it would be difficult. "Cleveth, you've got to come," Liza says. During the ensuing pause, I imagine that Cleveth explains that it is ten o'clock and she isn't sure she can get from Canarsie in Brooklyn to our house. Liza repeats emphatically, "*Cleveth, you've got to come.*" When Cleveth replies, Liza relaxes and hands the phone back to me.

I hold it to my ear. "Hi, Cleveth."

"Phil, I don't know if I can get there, but I'll try. I think one of my sons can bring me."

Molly becomes restless. I go to her and say, "I can see that you want Mommy. But since she is busy with Lizie, is there anything I can do to help you, sweetie?"

She shakes her head and turns away, almost huffing to her room, leaving me feeling helpless and frustrated. I turn to nestle with Elena and Liza. After a moment, Elena suggests that I go after Molly. *Are you kidding?* I think. *I just made my best try to reach out to Molly and*—I allow my face to show my disagreement. I am prepared to settle down in front of them, until Liza, speaking slowly and with labored breath, adds her opinion: "Daddy, I think ... you should try ... one ... more ... time."

Okay, wise child. I cannot refuse her.

Helena decides that it is time for her to leave. It is late, and she has done all she can to ease Liza's discomfort. She will keep in touch by phone. I show her to the door on the way up to Molly's room.

I take a few deep breaths before I knock. She is lying on her bed, tense and unhappy. "Can I talk with you, Mol?" She grudgingly assents. "What's bothering you, sweetie?"

"I don't get any time with Mommy. I know she has to help Lizie, but I still feel bad about it."

"How about if you tell Mommy that you want some time with her whenever it is possible? Even if you can't get what you want, you will have tried. It seems more likely to get you what you want than stomping off." Molly nods that this is a good idea. "I know you haven't had enough time with Mommy, but are you also upset at not having enough time with Lizie? I'm upset at seeing Lizie dying. Aren't you?" Molly seems to relax as she murmurs agreement. On a hunch, I ask her, "What did you hear Liza say to you?"

" 'We think it's time I'm going to die.' "

"Yes, but what else?"

"Nothing."

"Did you hear her tell you 'I just want you to know that I really love you'?"

Molly's face softens. "I didn't hear her say that to me. I heard her say something like that to Cleveth on the phone."

"A lot was going on, but she said that to you, bean." She looks immensely relieved and her mood lightens. We talk more easily about the strain of wanting to be close to Liza and to her mother.

Molly acknowledges that it is awful to see Liza so uncomfortable. "She can't breathe, she doesn't even want to be touched, except only a little bit by Mommy. It's like she's fading away."

"She is," I agree. Molly's eyes well up. She lets me give her a hug and returns it strongly. I ask her if she wants to go back downstairs with me. She nods. There, I sit beside Liza and Elena. Molly sits nearby, watching.

Liza is still. Her eyes are sometimes open, sometimes drifting shut or at half-mast. Elena holds her gently, her arms lightly on Liza's sides. From time to time, she bestows gentle touches of affection, careful not to offer more contact than Liza wants. Nanny rests on the brown couch, but she gets up and leaves periodically, needing to cry and wanting to do so privately.

After a few minutes, Molly walks in front of Liza and asks for her attention. "I love you, Lizie," Molly mumbles. Unable to hear her, Liza asks Molly what she said. Bravely, Molly repeats herself, first as a louder mumble, then clearly and audibly. "I love you, Lizie." Liza's face lights up with a small smile, there is the subtlest lift of her puffy cheeks. She extends her arms and the girls hug. Elena and I have tears in our eyes.

Cleveth arrives around midnight, with one of her sons and daughters-in-law. Liza, aware of her presence, rouses herself to say, "Hi, Cleveth." Gasping and nauseated, Liza won't let Cleveth touch her. But with a gesture of her arm and the murmured word "Here," she indicates that she wants Cleveth to sit by her left knee, within the little nest around Liza. Quietly, Liza says, "Cleveth, you don't have to bathe me anymore." Through her tears, Cleveth tells Liza that she loves her. Other than that, we speak little. Love and distress, love and heartache, fill the air. After an hour, Cleveth leaves.

Elena and I reassure Liza that it is okay for her to let go and that our love for her will never end.

Around 1:30 a.m., Liza begins to retch. She asks Elena to stand up and hold her so as to ease the retching and nausea. Elena gives herself to this completely. I call Helena, and she directs me to give Liza more IV medicine. After disposing of the syringe, I walk back to them.

Liza has stopped retching. She rests her head on her mother's shoulder. I circle my arms around them both. Nanny Charlotte and Molly sit together nearby. Liza murmurs, "Now." She goes limp. Her eyes close. She continues to gasp, though more slowly. Deeply in coma. She is going.

Elena and I, crying, hold each other and Liza. Gently, we put her down on the sofa, at her spot. Then Charlotte and Molly and Elena and I take turns holding Liza on our laps.

After everyone has taken the time they need with Liza, Elena and I decide to take her upstairs to our bedroom so that we can try to get some rest. She droops like a sack of potatoes. In her limpness, it is harder for us to carry her. Molly holds her head, I hold her chest, Lainie holds her legs. We do our best to hold on to her body, not to let her head or limbs flop awkwardly. When we get to our bed and put Liza down on her back, Lainie and Molly go back downstairs to say good night to Nanny. Listening to Liza's gasping breath, it occurs to me that she could choke on her own secretions—which might be horrible to hear and for Liza to feel, if she can still experience her body. On my own, I roll her over to lie facedown. As I try to flatten her, she seems to stiffen and raise herself eerily. I push out at the creases of her arms to bend her elbows. Bizarrely, when one arm bends, the other straightens. It is an absurd moment. Finally, I get both of her arms bent, and her body feels like it is relaxing. But when I stand up, her arms straighten again, and her torso pops up, almost into a crawling position. I thought she was far beyond words, but I hear her utter, "Can't do that." Flabbergasted, I call to Elena and tell her what I heard. Changing strategy, we construct a hillock of pillows. Together we turn Liza over and prop up her body, which is again fully limp.

Elena gets into bed and moves behind Liza, keeping her pledge to hold Liza while she is dying. I nestle beside both of them. Molly falls asleep at the foot of our bed. Nanny sleeps downstairs in Elena's office. Occasionally, we speak of our love for Liza and for one another. We continue to weep. Liza's breathing labors on, rasping, deep, slow, and long. Elena and I drift in and out of sleep. It seems that I have just finished listening to a handful of breaths, but each time I notice the clock, I see that another hour or two has passed.

At dawn, when Elena gets up to use the bathroom, I hold Liza. I realize that I yearn to keep holding her. Helena calls, and Elena talks to her before getting back into bed. I tell Elena that I want to share holding Liza with her. She lies down next to me, and we form a V with our bodies, within which Liza rests upon us both. Behind Liza, we hold each other.

Liza's loud, stridorous breaths slow. Pauses and occasional gasps interrupt the strained rhythm. Helena arrives, Charlotte lets her in. Carrying a tray of syringes filled with various medicines, Helena moves to our bedside. As she finds and uncaps the end of Liza's Broviac, Molly stirs and watches. Over a short period, Helena administers most of the medicines on the tray. Every few minutes, she pauses to listen to Liza, who is breathing more erratically. Then, with one extended, huge, gurgly, groan-like expiration, Liza's breathing stops.

We continue to hold her for a few minutes.

After a bit, Elena says, "I want to wash her." Shira once mentioned that washing the newly dead was an old custom. It feels right.

Helena offers, "Shall I remove the Broviac?"

"Please do," I say. Quickly, with surprising ease, Helena removes it. Then Molly and I undress her. We give Liza her last sponge bath. I have the irrational notion of wanting to make Liza's body more comfortable, so I push on her bladder; her urine fills a towel.

The three of us finish bathing her. Elena picks a strong red matching top and bottom adorned with a picture of Jasmine from Disney's *Aladdin* to put on Liza's body—an outfit she loved. Molly, Elena, and I maneuver Liza into the red set, and we carry her back downstairs.

We lay her down on the long sofa. We sit with her, each in turn and in pairs and all together, Molly, Nanny, Elena, and I. We try to grasp that this dear body betrayed our child, sister, grandchild. We try to understand that Liza is dead. We touch her hair, her skin. Molly explores her in the most free and natural way—touching, caressing, squeezing. She feels the special places she always loved to touch— Liza's ear, her earlobes, the edge of her ears, the rubbery parts. I do so too. We look under her lids at her eyes and in her mouth.

We call the funeral home. They will take Liza's body first to the hospital for an autopsy, then to the funeral home, and after the service, to the crematorium. We ask them to wait until midday so that we can sit beside Liza's body for some hours longer. We call Aunt Lisa and Grandma Doris and Cleveth, and shortly they come over. We sit around Liza's body. Occasionally, I get up and come back to see that Liza has not moved. Is this red-clad body Liza or only Liza's body? *Where is Liza?* I wonder. *Where is Liza's spirit?* I sob again. With Liza's rasping breath now absent, we fill the air with wailing, crying, sobbing, sighing, and, every so often, as Liza often requested, a few minutes of silence.

❋   ❋   ❋

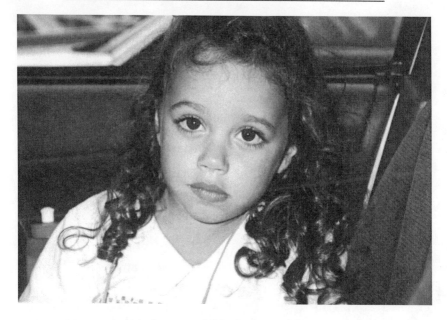

A short good life, Summer 1994.

When the two morticians arrive, they efficiently, anonymously, and respectfully don rubber gloves, come to the couch, and unfold a white plastic bag with a zipper down the side, like a garment bag. Into it they slip Liza's cooling, stiffening body. They bring a wheeled stretcher to the floor beside the couch and lift Liza's bagged body onto it. They roll her down the hall. We walk with them, not only to hold open the doors, but to accompany Liza's body. We stand on the stoop of our building, watching as they carry her down the steps. They place the bag into the back of their vehicle. They get in and drive away. I have the urge to wave.

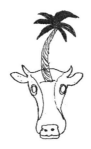

Epilogue:
Through Loss, Deeper Hues

2019

I Have Blue

When he was three and a half, I took Solomon on our first camping trip. He sat in a car seat in the back with a finger puppet of Blue from the show *Blue's Clues* on the forefinger of his right hand, while Magenta occupied the forefinger of his left.

"Blue, Daddy and I are going camping this weekend; nobody else is coming." My ears open wide, eager to hear Blue's rejoinder. None comes.

"Blue, Daddy and I are going camping this weekend; nobody else is coming." Silence.

Aha! Dimly, it dawns on me that I am to participate. As Blue. "Really, Solomon? Where's everybody else?"

"Well, Molly is visiting her friend Sandy, who is having her bat mitzvah party this weekend, and Mommy is preparing for a talk she is going to give and is spending some time with Aunt Lisa."

"So that's the family?"

"Well, I have a sister Liza, but she died."

"Really, Solomon? What happened?"

"She got leu-kee-me-a, and she died."

"Oh my, Solomon, I'm sorry. That's very sad."

"Yeah, life's like that."

I believe I was mute for a bit after that, wondering what a phrase like that could mean to my son at this age.

I have the little Blue on my desk—two dark blue eyes and a dark blue nose like a jigsaw puzzle piece, big jowls, ears merrily akimbo, and little pink tongue. Putting Blue on my finger, I look at him. What is this expression? Curiosity, expectancy, receptivity, wonder? And what has become of Magenta?

Should a Child Know?

Whether to inform a terminally ill child that she will die is a decision that must be weighed carefully. Historically, health care workers have avoided telling bad news, and I am glad to know that trends are changing.

Sometimes the team of helpers favors being direct with a child, and the parents object, wanting the child to be protected. I consulted with several families with a terminally ill child. In one frequent scenario, one or both parents insist that everyone act happy and upbeat at all times. All talk of illness is banned, and any talk of illness is in a context of believing that there would be a cure, even if by miracle. If the parents are of one mind, the child may feel forced to play a role so as to support his parents' pretense. If only one parent holds this position, there is sure to be a painful rift between them. It often seems that they are fighting to deny the reality at hand. And the child is caught up in their struggle.

One parent articulated that she kept her painful and sad feelings to herself, but succeeded at compartmentalizing them, locking them down. I said that it sounded like a rather lonely way to navigate. And I wondered whether her son might be similarly in a lonely place, full with worry about what lay ahead and with no one to speak to, no one with whom he could openly discuss his worries or questions. The intervention was salutary; when she rested with her son that night, she said that she welcomed anything he might say or ask, happy or sad. With obvious relief, the boy said he knew he was dying, and they wept together.

I believe that for Liza, knowing that she was dying allowed her to come to grips with the situation in a breathtaking way, to say good-bye to us, to prepare herself for death with immense dignity and grace. Sharing the understanding of her approaching death allowed us all to share a depth of love and closeness unlike any I had ever known before. That love sustained us when she died, and in a fundamental way, it sustains us still.

The Meaning of Words

I read to Solomon many of the books I once read to Liza. Like Liza, he interrupted my reading to ask about unfamiliar words.

"What does 'luckily' mean?" he asked.

Did she ask about "luckily"? I wondered. I used to know the words she asked about. I used to remember some of my explanations, some of the known words to which she compared the new one. I hated not being able to remember. What could I tell him about luck?

"Luck is how we speak of something happening for no reason we know. If the thing that happens is good, we call it lucky. If bad, unlucky."

"Like Ojo the Unlucky!" Solomon recalled from one of the Oz stories I read to both of them. Frequently, he brings her to my mind, and an instant later he circles her, eclipses her, with his own curiosity, energy, and humor—similar, but distinct and unique.

Once when I read to Solomon at bedtime, he interrupted with so many questions, so many excited ideas about what might be about to happen in the story, it got to be time for bed after reading only a few pages. I felt myself becoming impatient with his questions, even while I knew that each was delicious. *Don't you know we need to read—Read—READ?* I almost asked him.

Counting

if they ask
how many children
do you have
I almost always know
how many I have
I'm ready to shout
or sing
or say

three not two
three
if they ask
how old she is
a simple question
I brought upon myself
I don't know what to say
how to add
six years alive and the time since
six plus one is usually seven
but now
I don't know what to say
how to count
for a long time
she was stuck stuck at six
but now she lies far beyond
any single rational number

Song of Solomon

Age five. At the street corner, when the lighted sign said DON'T WALK, I stopped, mindful of being with my son, and he is learning from me, and I want him to learn stopping, to stay safe. While waiting, holding hands, he tugged on mine and asked, "Why didn't they work?"

"Solomon, what didn't work? What are you—?"

"Why didn't the medicines work?" he asked.

"That is such a good question, Solomon. Unfortunately, I don't know why they didn't work. Sometimes they do, and sometimes they don't, and we don't understand a lot about why they do or don't. I wish I knew too."

"Ummmm." He made some noise of comprehension.

"You have a lot going on in there." I ruffled his hair. "Keep your questions comin'."

"Okay."

By now, we'd missed the light, waited for the next WALK.

✻ ✻ ✻

A few weeks later, again walking down the street, Sol hummed, as he often did, but this time he stopped and turned to me.

"Did you hear what I was humming?"

"Yeah."

"I'm making up a song."

"That's cool," I said. He'd never made up a song before as far as I knew.

"It's a song for Liza. The first part," and he reprised humming the first part. "That's the happy part, cuz we're happy that the medicine worked for two years. And the second part," and he reprised the second part, with tones lower and slower. "That's the sad part, cuz we're sad she died."

"That's wonderful, boy!"

"Can we write it down?"

"Of course. When we get home later, we can sit with the piano and figure out the notes and write them down on music paper."

And when we got home later, he hummed for Elena, and they did peck at the piano and transcribe his song for his sister.

Not Invisible Children

Molly told me about the "invisible children" of northern Uganda, abducted, murdered, terrorized, and enlisted into an army of child soldiers by Joseph Kony. When Molly sent me the link, I watched the video on my computer screen and pledged financial support. When I showed Solomon, he insisted that he contribute some of his weekly allowance as well. After Elena watched it, we all participated in a consciousness-raising rally called "The Rescue."

Stepping back, I am struck by the sequence. With our support, Molly ventured into the world, in search of meaning and healing. Sensitive to the plight of children facing horror, she shared with us her experience teaching English to the children of Ethiopia. She shared what she'd learned about the children of central Africa, making the otherwise invisible children visible. Inspired by Molly, we find our way to a new vision of a much wider world moving forward—all of it is part of Liza's legacy.

The Sofa

it is time to replace the sofa
our embarrassing sofa
our guest gave the final signal
toying with the frayed fabric
mindlessly enlarging the hole

through which the wooden frame
which should never be seen
could be seen
and that was after he moved over
from the seat where he sank
too low down to be comfortable
intuiting what we know
of the spring
that has broken through the bottom
and now pushes into the floor
but
but
this is the original sofa on which she sat
on which she slept on which
she played the bakery games the tickling games
the drive away on vacation games
this is the merry sofa on which she jumped
while singing the silly birthday songs
(that we looked like a monkey
and we smelled like one too)
this is the charmed sofa on which she sat us
to perform with her sister
The Show—
whatever that week's show might be
skits or jokes, dances or tricks
by the pair of little hams
this is the same solid sofa on which she sat rooted
taking pills of all sorts
having blood infused or removed
having creams rubbed in
having deep muscle massage or the lightest tickling
from which she cried in agony
and on which she slept
lost in narcotic
too deep for too long
this is the safe sofa that was her base
from which to face her dwindling days
from which to declare her love and say goodbye
it is the soiled sofa
on which she wheezed and puked
and breathed her last
it is the hated place
where we sat with her
when she was dead
and sat by her
when she was still
until they came and bagged her body
and now
it is the dreadful vacated sofa

where on those she trusted
she leaned heavily
and where when I sit
when I lie back
I feel her

I imagine her finding out about
the new sofa—a sumptuous gorgeous cobalt blue
I can almost hear the quick patter of her feet
dashing down the hall
to celebrate
I can hear her squeal of joy
as she flings herself and flies
into its cushions
the Ultrasuede texture
the smell of its newness
the color she knows why we chose

Something I'd Like to Share

One of the psychiatrists in my office suite, Dan, was a priest and a doctor. At one point early in Liza's illness, he offered in a heartfelt way, "If there's anything I can ever do to help, let me know."

Lucid at that moment, I thanked him and then added, "Simply ask me how Liza is doing from time to time; that would be a great help."

"Of course I will."

But in the following two years, even when Liza was dying, he never asked about her. One day, not long after Liza died, amid a discussion about the paper towels and toilet paper we were buying for the office, I noticed that I was upset, far more than I had ever been about paper products.

I went to him later in the day. "I realize that I was getting much too angry earlier. It's about something else. Do you realize you never asked about Liza?" There was a still and charged moment between us.

"I know," he said immediately, flushing. "I'm sorry. I've never been able to deal with death."

I was flabbergasted. I knew from my own firsthand experience in medical school that doctors might never become comfortable dealing with death. Ironically, while almost every medical student delivers a baby, they may never engage with a dying patient. But I had a fantasy that every priest must be trained to deal with death. Suddenly, I saw the flaw in my reasoning. Just as we expect doctors to be prepared to deal with death, I had foisted my own hopes on this man because he was a priest.

When I told Elena about the encounter, she joked, "I'd better be careful talking with you about paper products!" She added with chagrin, "It had to be something like that, didn't it?"

Yes, it had to be something like that. We don't do a good job of dealing with death, with dying, with trauma, with suffering. And Dan is not the only one who vanished, apparently it being too much, too painful to stay near. My friend Jon did too. Perhaps there is some resonance between them and the medical student who was so restless, so inclined to leave the Day Zero talk, as I imagined him. In that way, I can see my own limitations too, like theirs. There have been times I haven't been able to comprehend standing in another's shoes—what it means to be severely disabled, to be addicted, to be transgender, to be abused, to be an abuser. All of these realities have been difficult for me to deeply imagine. But less difficult now. And what is the difference? The difference is that during the course of our journey with Liza, we witnessed her capacity to grow, the capacity to stay openhearted in the face of extreme suffering. To stay loving.

And in receiving our support, and giving hers, she nurtured our capacities to do the same.

If she'd survived, is there any doubt that she'd have been a force for all those she met, a wellspring for expanding such capacities, for stepping toward our best selves? If she'd learned of other children who did not have the privilege of access to excellent health care, what would she have said and done? If she'd learned about racism and oppression and inequity and police brutality—if her life had included knowledge of and exposure to such atrocities—I imagine she would have been incensed, would have cared deeply.

Only after Liza died did I read the work of eloquent author and AIDS activist Paul Monette. I imagine telling Liza about some of his last words: "Go without hate, but not without rage; heal the world."

As I understand her, she'd have brought energy for healing the world. I hope that despite her short life, she still can. And that is why it was important for me to write about her life, not just to heal myself, but importantly, to share her courageous spirit.

Once I cooled down and forgave my office suitemate for his neglect, I imagine talking to Liza about it as if she were here. Yes, I do have her with me in spirit. *We know what to do*, she'd say. *Let's go talk with him. Give him one good try.*

So with Liza guiding me, I'd say to Dan or Jon or Phil or Barb:

It's hard for almost all of us to deal with death. But we have to change that. Especially for healers, but equally for each of us. Let's set aside some time. I'll tell you a story about our experience with Liza.

It changed me. It was crushing and at times left me feeling broken. But it has broken me open. There was so much beauty in it. I learned how much we have to give one another, how much we can lift and love one another by tuning in to loss, not dodging it.

It's true that Liza's life was too short, but in a way, no matter how many years we have, life is too short for us all. She's not the only one to suffer, but she's the one I know well, the one who opened my eyes. Can I tell you about her? It will change you, too. For the better. Trust me. If you wish, you can carry her too. There is enough for everyone.

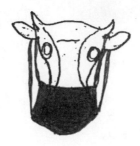

ACKNOWLEDGMENTS

M y mother instilled in me a love of reading and writing, a respect for words well written. And from there, it was an easy step to feel called to try to find the right ones to catch hold of personal history and to shrink the gap between the buzz of experience and the words with which to capture it. I love that undertaking.

Yet I've had to contend with a potent part of myself that snickered, *You? Write?* It's taken a lot of work to free myself of the torment and inhibition of that doubting voice. Many helpers have assisted me thus far: Leonard Diamond, Ben Cirlin, Shira Ruskay, Linda Smith, Ricki Bernstein, and Annie and Michael Mithofer. And I have enjoyed mentorship in writing from Lenora DeSio, Gladden Shrock, and Hugh Burgess. Joe Spieler traveled a long part of this journey with me and invited me to link the present with the past; finding me try and fail, resist and flail, he pressed me again. Thank you. I am grateful to have you all with me!

When I completed a draft of the book, I had not considered making a book proposal. Such a marketing tool seemed silly to me, backward. Thanks to Stephen Wesley, who helped me see the wisdom, at times, of playing by the rules and teaching them to me. He guided me in crafting the proposal, which helped me find McFarland. Ted Kaupf provided the introduction to his contact at McFarland. Cindy Nixon edited my final draft with the relentlessness of the best dental hygienist, bringing to my attention every blemish, inconsistency, overused word, and errant comma. However, unlike any dental hygienist I've known, she was a hoot to work with—fun, fast, and wonderful.

Even with all of that assistance, I would have faltered without the encouragement of many friends and students, some of whom read pieces and drafts as this project evolved. Specifically, I want to thank Pilar Jennings, Laura Palmer, and Chip Insinger for their stewardship. I am grateful for the added encouragement of Jules and Susan Kerman, Lorraine Anastasio, Nate Kravis, Rohn Friedman, Katharine Muir, Ted Scovell, Emily Nash, Valerie Linet, Alan Bernstein, Gita Vaid, Larry Shaderowfsky, Jon Belford, Alan Barasch, Jon Polan, Chip Brown, Dawn Drzal, Judy Gallent, Lisa Rubin, and Gary Singer. Anne Nelson commented in a manner that I could hear, "You can write."

Joe Fins, Bob and Amy Pollack, Nancy Hutton and Larry Wissow, Suzanne Garfinkle, John M. Saroyan, Bob Maki, Anne Ulanov, Susan Coates, Burt Lerner, and Herb Bernstein expressed belief in the value of Liza's story by giving me opportunities to speak to various medical and academic audiences. Those experiences helped me to hone what it was that I wanted to share and say.

In my most fear-addled younger years, I shunned groups. Since Liza died, though, fear has lessened. I've engaged in many groups, and they have enriched me enormously. I hardly recognize myself. I feel as though the members of these groups have extended their hands and put them gently to my back, helping me to persevere. These include the self-dubbed Best Group (for study of using EMDR with children) formed around Colette Linnihan, with Jill Kristal, Erica Fross, Josie Diaz, Amarilis Rivera, Michael Clifford, and Eric Beers; an SE (somatic experiencing) experiential group initiated by Roger Saint-Laurent and Peter Taylor and continuing with Rachel Ravin, Leslie Gibson, Nina Allred, Vartika Mutha, and Jess Linick. A writing workshop helped me reconsider every decision I made with this manuscript, and for that, I am grateful to Gerry Jonas, Rob Bates, Patrick Burhenne, Bob Heller, Malcolm Mitchell, and Jane Stark. Most recently, I have enjoyed the embrace of the community of friends and colleagues at MAPS (the Multidisciplinary Association of Psychedelic Studies), with whom I have been working for the past several years, foremost among them Ingmar Gorman, Willa

Hall, Casey Paleos, Sarah Robinson, Alex Belser, Emily Horowitz, Jill Silverman, and Elizabeth Nielson.

I introduced you to Colleen, Carolyn Fein, Peter Steinherz, and Nancy Kerman—all of whom cared for Liza and our family with deep compassion and intelligence. There were so many more who lifted us up, so many nurses and nurses' aides, escorts and housekeepers, radiology techs, even the man whose car I jumped into who drove me to the hospital. Thank you for your kindness. I can see you in my mind, but I don't know all your names. I remember you, though, and I am grateful that you showed me how much we have to offer one another. I strive to do likewise.

Of all the encouragers, none come close to Molly, Liza, and Solomon, who might hear of a challenge I face—a fitness goal or the quest to finish and publish this book, for example. I hear their unhesitant, spirited, optimistic declaration: *You can do it, Daddy!* Remembering Liza's sage advice that I "try one more time" infuses me with fortitude.

In that spirit, I must disclose that when I listened to music while writing and rewriting, of greatest value were Southern Avenue's "Don't Give Up" and Glenn Gould's "So You Want to Write a Fugue?" I'd listen to them on auto-replay and slide into the zone of timelessness. Remembering this, I envision my father, Liza, all of my allies beaming. Go ahead and write it I did.

Above all, Elena. For her, I'll borrow from Viktor Frankl: "I grasped the meaning of the greatest secret that human poetry and human thought and belief have to impart: The salvation of man is through love and in love." In our joys and sorrows, Elena discovered this alongside me. She read every word and version of this book. What can I say? When I see her face, when I hold her hand, I am home.

INDEX